THE GLOW CODE

THE GLOW CODE

A Cheat Sheet for Feeling, Looking, and Being Your Best at Any Age

MICHELLE McIVOR

ROWMAN & LITTLEFIELD
Lanham • Boulder • New York • London

Published by Rowman & Littlefield
An imprint of The Rowman & Littlefield Publishing Group, Inc.
4501 Forbes Boulevard, Suite 200, Lanham, Maryland 20706
www.rowman.com

86-90 Paul Street, London EC2A 4NE

British Library Cataloguing in Publication Information available

Library of Congress Cataloging-in-Publication Data available
ISBN 978-1-5381-8072-3 (pbk : alk. paper)
ISBN 978-1-5381-8073-0 (ebook)

∞™ The paper used in this publication meets the minimum requirements of American National Standard for Information Sciences—Permanence of Paper for Printed Library Materials, ANSI/NISO Z39.48-1992.

In memory of my grandmothers,
Florence Magnan and Adaliane Bethune,
who showed me what it means to age well

NOTHING BUT GRATITUDE

THIS BOOK WOULD NOT HAVE BEEN POSSIBLE WITHOUT THE many experts, maverick thinkers, and trailblazers who agreed to share their time, wisdom, and advice with me for the sake of my readers. I am beyond grateful.

As you'll read in the following pages, they are brilliant and generous, funny and kind. I hope you'll consider following them on social media, subscribing to their newsletters, listening to their podcasts, and buying their books. Because their insights will change your life. I know that because they've changed mine. With that, I give a heartfelt thank-you to everyone whose genius helped shape *The Glow Code*, listed here in alphabetical order:

Tina Alster

Ashton Applewhite

Diane Berson

Suzanne Blons

Bianca Bosker

Lori Brotto

Karen B.K. Chan

Eldo Ray Estes

Vivien Fam

Marisa G. Franco

Jennifer Gaudiani

Megan Golightly

Shelby Harris

Nadia Hrkac

Summer Innanen

Stacey Irvine

Lisa Kellett

Liz Layton

Margo Maine

Jill Margo

Jennifer Martin

Michelle McGrattan

Crystal Mckenzie

Myka Meier

Shasta Nelson

Russell Poldrack

Brigid Schulte

Krista Scott-Dixon

Julie Shipley-Strickland

Susan Silk

Stacy Sims

Abbie Smith-Ryan

Helen Tansey

Fatima Thomas

Reagan Wetherill

Tamar Zenith

Janet Zuccarini

CONTENTS

INTRODUCTION

I FOUND MY FIRST GRAY EYEBROW HAIR A FEW MONTHS AGO. Correction: My first gray eyebrow hair proudly announced itself a few months ago. Seemingly overnight, it had sprouted from my face as if to say, "Hello, world, I'm heeeere!"

I was less enthused.

Of course, I saw this hair when I could do nothing, zilch, nada about it. I'd just dropped my kids off at daycare and was stopped at a red light, glancing at my reflection in the rear-view mirror. And there it was—a long, coarse, gray hair jutting out at an odd angle from the inner corner of my left eyebrow, glimmering in the sunlight. Couldn't it at least get in line with the rest of my brow? The audacity of this hair!

That's when two things really hit me: (1) Despite my best attempts to stay youthful, I am aging—and there's no hiding it. And (2) Why don't I always keep a set of tweezers in my car?!

For the rest of the day, I was sure everyone I met with was staring at my errant eyebrow hair. I couldn't wait to get home to pluck the damn thing. When I eventually did later that night—and by eventually, I mean the minute I walked through the door—I was so relieved.

A few weeks passed. I didn't think about it again.

And then the second gray hair popped up.

That's when I started to Google things like "Does plucking gray hair make more grow?" and "Can you dye eyebrows?"

and "Am I having more or less sex with my husband than the national average?"

That last question was unrelated, but it had been on my mind. And if you're curious, the answers were no, yes, and more. Yay us.

Why am I telling you all this? Because if you're a woman—or you just care about how you're aging!—and, like me, you're brushing up against midlife, chances are we share the same types of concerns, questions, and Google searches.

Have you wanted to drink less alcohol but not give it up? Me too. Wondering if you really need to take a multivitamin, a handful of supplements, and that pricey collagen powder? Great question. Interested in switching your decades-old makeup routine because you're now a woman in your forties with crow's feet and puffy eyes? Same, girl. Same.

But where do we even begin? And more importantly, who has the time to sort through all the information and products at our disposal? I feel overwhelmed with my life at the best of times, let alone when I'm perusing the aisles in Sephora.

That's because navigating life as a woman between the ages of 35 and 50 is no joke. We have less time to ourselves but more concerns to deal with, ranging from the big to the small. When I turned 40, lines dug in around my eyes and mouth. My body fat percentage crept up even though I had lost weight. I had a hard time sleeping through the night. My lower back started to hurt more. So did some of my friendships.

Worst of all, I couldn't escape the sneaky suspicion that I should have learned how to deal with these matters by now. I was a grown woman, after all, and not getting any younger. What had I been doing with my life? I should have prepared for this! I should have known better!

See, at 44, I am well past the glory days of my youth, if you consider going to the bar four nights a week "glorious." I have a wonderful husband and two kids. A mortgage. A job to pay said mortgage. By all accounts, I am an adult. But despite being told repeatedly that I was having "geriatric" pregnancies at the tender ages of 36 and 38—thanks so much for that confidence boost, docs—I am years away from becoming a senior. And I feel like there's so much I still don't know.

If you're at this stage, too, I don't need to tell you about the myriad of questions that run through my brain when I can't sleep at night.

Whatever, let me tell you anyway.

I wonder things like: Does collagen powder prevent wrinkles? Are skinny jeans and side parts ever coming back in style? How am I supposed to get in five hours of exercise a week? I barely have time to shower! When I do workout, should I focus on cardio or weights? Which bottle of wine should I bring to dinner on Friday night? Does everyone else own art? Should I? Why can't I fall back asleep at night? Do I need to use a face serum? What kind? Am I a good friend?

Let's just say it's not a small list of concerns.

Thankfully, chatting about them with my girlfriends has made me realize I am not alone. We have spent many wine-fuelled evenings discussing such things, helping each other as best we can. We've shared info we've read in magazines or seen on TikTok or heard in passing, all in hopes of sorting out what's true, what works, and what doesn't. Because, I mean, aging: We're all in it together. And we all want answers.

In this book, that's exactly what you're going to get.

My name is Michelle McIvor and, aside from being a woman who's heading into her mid-forties at full speed, I've been a journalist for nearly twenty years. So, when I became hyper-focused on aging—and aging like a superwoman, no less—I decided to reach out to the experts, trailblazers, and maverick thinkers who could answer our burning questions about aging, cut through the fads and trends, and arm us with the credible, practical advice we deserve.

How did I decide who to speak with? Well, being a reporter for many years has given me a good radar for bullshit. On the flip side, I've learned which kind of voices can be trusted: researchers who've published peer-reviewed studies, doctors and dermatologists who come pre-vetted from organizations such as the American Academy of Dermatology, subject matter experts with verifiable credentials, and often-quoted authorities who appear in fact-checked publications. Those are all top-notch people to chat with. And that's who I've tapped for our purposes.

The first person I reached out to was Dr. John Berardi, co-founder of the world's largest nutrition coaching and education company, Precision Nutrition. John is one of the most trusted voices in wellness and, for many years, was my go-to interviewee for all things nutrition. But you won't find John in this book. Instead, you'll find a few of the female researchers, authors, and scientists he pointed me to, such as Dr. Stacy Sims. Stacy is a former Stanford researcher who's passionate about studying women's unique physiology and maximizing their athletic abilities. In John's words, "She wrote this generation's definitive book on what women need to do differently than men with exercise and nutrition." Speaking with her and some of his other suggested interviewees gave me an excellent starting point for this book.

But for most of my interviews, I reached out directly to experts I'd found, researched, and vetted online, seen quoted as credible sources in major media outlets, or followed on social media for their distinct brand of genius. I told them I had burning questions about how all of us gals can age well.

Sure enough, they had answers galore.

That's what you'll find in this book, grouped by topic like skincare, fitness, and friendships and packaged into digestible, actionable pieces of advice you can put to work today.

Now, I didn't want to just dump a bunch of information on you and wish you luck. No, ma'am. That would make for a dull read. And as we've discussed, life is too short—and full and distracting—for that kind of book. To keep things a bit spicy, I'm sharing what happened when I put the experts' advice to work in *my* life.

And it's been a wild ride.

Over the course of this book-writing journey, I've thrown out most of my skincare products. Reached out to an old friend to rekindle our relationship. Gently eased away from another. Curbed my drinking. Rethought everything from how I apply my eyeliner to why I exercise. Incorporated two nutritional supplements into my daily routine. Learned not only which vibrator works best during sex, but which product enhances my orgasms.

Apologies if that last one caught you off guard. When you get to the sex chapter, you and your vagina will thank me. So will your partner.

Along the way, I've spoken with the likes of Dr. Tina Alster, an acclaimed dermatologist, professor, and author; Fatima Thomas, a renowned makeup artist; Bianca Bosker, sommelier and author of the *New York Times* bestseller *Cork Dork*; Dr. Marisa Franco, the friendship expert and bestselling author; Dr. Abbie Smith-Ryan, an exercise physiologist, sports nutritionist, and prolific researcher; and Karen B.K. Chan, an award-winning sex and intimacy educator.

And following their advice has led to some astounding results. As in, I have never worked out less in my life and I'm getting stronger. Is that even possible? My friends drag me to my bathroom to see what products I'm using to get my glowing skin. And my husband wants to have a third kid. Joking! But he is always up for the practice sessions. (Sorry, but not sorry.)

In short, I wanted a cheat sheet for aging well that worked, so I made one. And now I'm sharing it with you.

Here's what this book will not do: shame you or make you feel bad about your life choices, like not wearing sunscreen for two full decades. Been there, done that, girl.

This book will also not feed you fluff, tell you to just think positively, or suggest you manifest your way to being the adult woman you'd love to be. I'm sharing real, practical advice, because I'm a geek about this stuff. I've written about women's health and wellness for years, but I've also read every article, blog post, and magazine story I can get my hands on. This book is for anyone else who will always click on the story titled "The 5 Skincare Products Dermatologists Swear By" or spend more than ten minutes watching Brooke Shields give a makeup tutorial on YouTube or have passionate conversations with girlfriends about what shoes to wear with wide-leg pants.

Here's what this book *will* do: give you actionable, credible advice that can make your life better and help you age well. It's comprehensive, yes, but don't worry about getting overwhelmed! I've distilled the important information down into one handy, easy-to-read guide you can trust. Think of it like this: If we poured truth serum over a stack of women's magazines, this information would come oozing out. We're tossing the misinformation and getting to the heart of what really works. Armed with this stellar info, my hope is you'll feel all lit up and inspired to make small changes that will yield big results.

On that note, I have a final thought to share. I know we're not supposed to care about certain things. We're supposed to be above it all. And, really, what's the point of even trying? According to society—and my obstetricians—we're old now. No longer sex symbols, just a bunch of geriatrics in the making.

Well, I say screw that.

We can be proud, strong women—the kind of women who are changing the world for good every day—and still want glowing skin in our forties and care about fashion trends and indulge our creative passions and try new things in the bedroom. That's the stuff that fills our days. It's real. It's grown up. And it matters.

We matter, and we deserve to have the life edits, habits, and strategies in this book at the ready. As you read *The Glow Code* to glean these golden nuggets of information, please don't feel tied to reading it front to back. Skip around. Choose your own adventure. Dig in where you're most curious. If you're a gal with minimum free time but maximum ambition to feel, look, and live better now, in midlife, and beyond, I hope you'll find this book helpful.

My ultimate wish is that you come away feeling great about your age, like the strong, creative, sexy, confident, smart woman you are. I want to feel that way, too, which is why I'm striving to embrace this stage of my life, gray eyebrow hairs and all. It's not always easy. But it's been a hell of a lot smoother knowing what I've learned while writing this book. This cheat sheet works, and I'm excited for you to give it a whirl.

Let's begin, shall we?

CHAPTER ONE

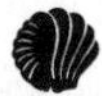

Build Muscle to Stay Fit, Maintain Your Strength, and Feel Like a Superwoman

I USED TO EXERCISE A LOT. SEE, I GREW UP IN A FAMILY THAT liked to move, be it tackling long hikes, strapping on our cross-country skis, or shooting hoops after dinner. In school, I played team sports, and then in college I learned to lift weights. No wonder I turned into an adult who loved getting a post-exercise high.

When I was young and carefree and had all the time in the world—yes, that would be my twenties and early thirties—I went to the gym to get it.

As you can probably guess, I spent most of my time doing what women raised in the '80s and '90s do: cardio. I'm one of those weirdos who enjoys sweaty cardio sessions, plus I'd always believed that doing long bouts of cardio was the best way to stay lean. I pushed myself hard, sprinting on the treadmill or running outside, and taking hour-long spin classes and boot camps. I also knew that lifting weights was important, obvi, so I'd take the odd strength class or run through a standard full-body routine using light to medium weights.

All told, I exercised four to five hours a week.

I look back on that now and all I can think is, *Oof, who's got that kind of time?!* Not me, at least anymore.

I can tell you the precise moment my fitness routine imploded: at 2:16 a.m. on September 26, 2016. That's when my first child, Hudson, shot from my vagina and into the world. Well, it was a lengthy, forceps-assisted birth that left me torn and sore for weeks, but you get the idea.

Having a kid was (duh) a massive change. Everything in my life was shaken up, every routine abandoned. I spent the first many months in a zombie-like state, sleep-deprived and foggy. Plus, I had to keep my boobs near my son. I was breastfeeding him and he was hungry, so getting outside the house was tricky. Getting to the gym? Impossible.

When I finally had enough energy (and a healed vagina), I needed to get back into exercise. My husband and I invested in a few sets of dumbbells, a weighted ball, and a small bench for me to use at home. I'd pull them out when Hudson napped—which, I swear, was never for longer than thirty minutes—and get a quick strength workout in.

For me, the biggest surprise wasn't that I loved working out at home. It was that my short workouts seemed to be as effective, if not more so, than what I'd been doing for years. Considering the only hour-long cardiovascular exercise I had was pushing the stroller around our neighborhood a few times a week, I felt fit and strong. And I liked how I looked in my clothes. It slowly dawned on me—I blame the brain fog for *how* slowly—that maybe fitness didn't have to eat up so much of my life.

Plus, I didn't have any other choice. Just twenty-two months after I had Hudson, my daughter Marlowe arrived. After three short pushes, she really *did* shoot from my vagina, which, as I needn't explain to any woman who's pushed a small human out of her body, was a pleasant and welcome surprise. Juggling two young kids with the demands of work, family, friends, and, uh, life meant I had even *less* time to exercise.

Sure, things eventually got easier. But just as I was ready to get outside of the house more—and renew my gym membership—COVID-19 hit. Given that my husband, kids, and I were now at home 24/7, and I still had to work and do all the things, I started to wonder: How much time do I really need to dedicate to exercise? What should I focus on now—weights or cardio? Am I going to die soon?

Strange, but a thought I'd been having. Being in a global pandemic didn't help, I'm sure, but in addition to blowing up my workout routine, having kids made me think a lot about dying. Specifically, how to avoid doing that. I had always exercised to feel and look good, but now the stakes were higher. When I looked at my kids' adorable little faces, my priorities shifted from feeling and looking good—which, don't get me wrong, I still wanted—to living a long, healthy, independent life.

But how?

Just as I was pondering how best to exercise and age well, one name started popping up on my Instagram feed: Stacy Sims, PhD. Respected health and wellness experts I follow were sharing her content—posts about exercise, nutrition, and the importance of getting *both* right as we age. When I saw her post telling menopausal women to "think LHS (Lift Heavy Shit) instead of LSD (Long Slow Distance)," I knew we had to chat. I'd only recently entered my forties, but menopause was a hop, skip, and handful of periods away, and I figured Stacy could tell me how to spend my precious exercise time.

Around the same time, Dr. John Berardi, the nutrition expert I've trusted for years, suggested I speak with Stacy for this book.

No wonder.

As an exercise physiologist, nutrition scientist, and former athlete, Stacy is one of the rare researchers dedicated to studying women's exercise performance potential and the nutrition we need to achieve it. She has directed research programs at institutions such as Stanford University and Auckland University of Technology, published more than seventy peer-reviewed papers, written or contributed to several books, and been named one of the top forty women changing the paradigm in her field, among other accomplishments. To sum up: She knows her stuff.

I started by reading all of Stacy's Instagram posts and her fantastic book for women called *Roar: How to Match Your Food and Fitness to Your Unique Female Physiology for Optimum Performance, Great Health, and a Strong, Lean Body for Life*. Next, I watched her TEDx Talk called "Women Are Not Small Men" (so good! also, how fit is she?!). And then, I sent her an email asking if we could chat.

That's how Stacy and I ended up on a video chat in the fall of 2021, she from the garage at her home in New Zealand (she needed a quiet space to chat because her 9-year-old daughter was at home) and me from our basement (I needed a quiet space because my kids were running wild upstairs).

Turns out, Stacy was just as excited to talk to me about aging.

"I take the Japanese viewpoint, which is that when you hit menopause, it's a new chapter of life and, all of a sudden, you're the wise one that everyone wants to come talk to," she told me. "I hate the western idea that depicts women as being old, decrepit, and useless. My mom's 75, and she and her husband have been out hiking Machu Picchu. My grandmother's 105 and she does push-ups against the wall every morning when she gets up. If you're taking care of your body and listening to it, then you can do stuff when you're 70 or 80."

According to Stacy, taking care of our bodies ultimately comes down to taking caring of our muscle. That's because well before we hit menopause, a biological state marked by twelve months of no periods, our body composition is changing. And not for the better. In the four to five years leading up to that point, research shows that women's body fat goes up while our bone mass and lean mass go down. We want to stop—and even reverse—that trend as soon as possible.

"You want to start building muscle mass *now* to avoid that really accelerated lean mass and bone loss that happens when you actually hit post-menopause," she says. "If you can stop the change in those early years, then you don't have as big of a worry afterward."

Thankfully, many things can help.

Following the existing recommendations isn't one of them.

"We know from the research that recommendations for 150 minutes of moderate-intensity activity counter what we should be doing," Stacy says. "It makes people fatter, slower, and tired." Those recommendations, according to Stacy, are not designed for active women who have plenty of untapped performance potential. She wants to help us tap into ours, so I asked her to rewrite the guidelines.

Here were her top three recommendations:

1. **Lift heavy, challenging weights two to three times per week.** It's the most effective way to maintain muscle, support bone health and stay mobile as we age. In fact, lifting heavy weights should be our number-one priority. "Women who don't [lift heavy] can expect to lose at least 3 percent of their muscle mass per decade after age 30," she says.

2. **Do two High-Intensity Interval Training (HIIT) sessions per week.** She recommends sprinting, biking, or rowing all-out at your maximal effort level for only twenty, thirty, or forty seconds at a time, with two to three minutes of rest in between each, ultimately stopping after ten intervals. And if you're new to this kind of workout, you can work up from two or three bursts. Either way, doing maximum-effort intervals reaps huge benefits. "Not only does it help with body composition and most aesthetic things women are looking for, but it increases bone density

and insulin sensitivity, and it helps keep that lean mass," she says. "It also helps with cognition and fatigue because it changes neuromuscular stimulation." Bye, brain fog.

3. **Eat a pre-workout snack with protein.** Consuming a small snack with protein before exercise is super beneficial, says Stacy, and having one after a long workout is essential, too. Whatever you do, though, don't exercise on an empty stomach. "When women train fasted and delay their food after, they stay in a breakdown state. That signals to the body there's not enough nutrition to support general health, as well as the stress of training," Stacy says. "The body reacts by slowing metabolism and muscle begins to waste away."

Yowza. I had been doing the exact opposite.

A few months into the pandemic, we bought a Peloton bike, so my cardio efforts were usually long and moderate, not short and intense. When I tackled the odd weights workout, I was using light weights—the same weights I'd used for years—as opposed to challenging myself. And I often exercised first thing in the morning or mid-afternoon, with no pre-workout snack to fuel me.

At least I'd been doing *one* thing right: not jumping on the intermittent fasting (IF) bandwagon. Frankly, the whole concept—alternating between lengthy periods of not eating and shorter periods of eating—never appealed to me because, well, I like to eat. And I especially like breakfast, which is a meal that typically gets nixed when you fast. But I've heard many women say that IF has helped them control calories and lose weight. In the short term, it might, Stacy says, but the long-term effects are terrible. "You might have good success for a few months but then you're wasting your muscle away and signaling your metabolism to slow down. We don't want that happening because we know with age your metabolism slows down anyway."

That's why IF is bad news for active women, although Stacy says it *can* be helpful for certain populations that may benefit from calorie restriction. It also seems to work better for men. "Most of the benefits we hear about intermittent fasting is based on male data," Stacy says. In women, though, IF triggers our bodies to stay in that "breakdown state" that not only destroys muscle mass but can lead to anxiety and depression. That's why eating throughout the day is a smart move. No objections here to that strategy!

As for correcting my wrongs, I told Stacy I was eager to incorporate pre-workout snacks and start lifting heavier weights, but I worried I'd waited too long. Was I screwed? Destined to be in a wheelchair at 70? She assured me it's never too late to change our ways.

She also assured me that women cannot—I repeat, cannot—get bulky from lifting heavy weights. "It's amazing women don't put precedence on lifting at all, but we've all grown up in that Jane Fonda, slow cardiovascular, long-distance, fat-burning shit. No one talked about lifting weights because you'd 'get too bulky,' but there's *no* research to show that women will get bulky," she says. "Even if you made no changes before you hit menopause other than putting an emphasis on lifting heavy, you'd see a massive amount of body composition change."

Dr. Abbie Smith-Ryan agrees.

"A woman is not going to look jacked unless she takes testosterone," she says. "We don't even get enough stimulus from the weights because we're always told to lift light!"

You might be thinking, "Okay, I hear ya. I'll try lifting heavier weights. Who's Abbie?"

Fair question.

Before I signed off with Stacy, all fired up to implement her advice and become the kind of woman who's crushing push-ups when she's 105, she suggested I chat with Abbie, a professor of exercise physiology at The University of North Carolina who runs a lab dedicated to finding the most feasible ways women can improve their fitness. She's also a sports nutritionist and a prolific researcher with over 165 peer-reviewed manuscripts. To sum up again: She knows her stuff.

I connected with Abbie via video chat and her enthusiasm for sharing advice for her fellow lady folk jumped through the screen. She was standing in her office as we chatted, visibly passionate about sharing her knowledge with us. "There are so many things that we can do to make aging feel so much better. And it doesn't have to be impossible! That's what motivates me as a scientist."

It also motivates her as a woman who wants to age well.

Abbie, who was a long-distance runner in college, is now in her late thirties, which means she grew up believing what we're all told as women—that cardio is best. She even held onto that belief while she was studying the opposite. But after years of researching what works best for women as they age—and applying it to her own life—she's a convert.

Today, she tackles the occasional long run for enjoyment but, à la Stacy Sims, she makes sure to get the *right* kind of cardio in every week. That means two HIIT workouts. "The best thing for women to do is support muscle mass. Cardiovascular exercise is good for your heart but not necessarily good for your muscles," she says. "But what we've found studying HIIT over the last decade is that it *can* build muscle, which most aerobic exercise cannot."

In addition to having faster effects on cardiometabolic health, HIIT also decreases insulin, helps with glucose stability, and is one of the best ways to burn more calories and fat post-exercise. Those effects support a greater change in body composition, fat use and metabolism—all things that mitigate some of the changes we see with age. The hardest part about HIIT? Letting go of the idea that our workouts must be long to be effective. "As a woman that was told to exercise for hours and knowing that tired feeling I get after running ten miles, when I'm done HIIT I feel like, 'Am I done?'" says Abbie. "It's ten minutes of work, essentially."

You read that right. Like Stacy, Abbie recommends ten intervals—but they're a minute-long each. After a brief warmup, you alternate between giving one minute of all-out effort and taking one minute off or easy, working up to ten sets of work. Including a five-minute warmup, it takes about twenty-five minutes total. The workout can be done at the gym on a treadmill, bike, or rower, or at home, whether you have that equipment on hand or head outside to run or tackle stairs. Abbie has studied this workout with many groups, including cancer survivors, people with knee osteoarthritis, and post-surgery patients. "In all those populations, it increases cardio-respiratory fitness, so it reduces risk for cardiovascular disease, and it builds muscle, which then supports metabolism. And it takes twenty minutes! I don't care who you are. You can do this workout."

Wondering how hard to work during the intervals? I did, too.

You might not like the answer.

"It should hurt a little bit," Abbie says, adding that you should pick an intensity and workload you could not sustain for a minute and twenty seconds. When you rest, you can come to a complete stop or keep your legs moving a bit. Just be warned you won't feel totally ready for that next interval. I can confirm it's less of an "I'm ready!" go-get-em-tiger type of feeling and more of a "Holy shit, another interval already?" breathless kind of muttering. But as Abbie says, that's exactly how HIIT should feel.

Doing HIIT twice a week will cover your cardio needs, she says. And if you can do it more than that, your intervals probably aren't intense enough.

To really focus on muscle mass, she too recommends lifting weights twice a week. The key? Doing fewer reps so that you can push yourself using heavier weights. "Most women are used to doing twelve to fifteen reps in a set with light weights. That's not as worth it," she says. "Now, something is better than nothing, but the best bang for your buck as a woman is to lift really heavy."

A common theme, no?

I asked Abbie to explain what lifting heavy looks like.

In some ways, it's a lot like HIIT. The workout she suggests is called High-Intensity Resistance Training, or HIRT, and, just like its cardio equivalent, it's quick, practical, and effective at building muscle. What makes it high intensity is lifting a heavy load and recovering for a short period.

Get Your HIRT On

The HIRT protocol that exercise physiologist Abbie Smith-Ryan recommends is simple, effective, and takes only 25 minutes to complete. The key to this workout is using weights so heavy you can only complete 6 to 8 reps in each set. When you can do 3 sets of 8, it's time to grab heavier weights. This progressive workout will challenge you, strengthen your whole body and, ultimately, help build muscle mass. Here's how to get it done:

1. Warm up however you like.
2. Do three sets of 6 to 8 reps each of the following exercises, resting for 20 to 30 seconds between each set and for 2.5 minutes before moving on to the next exercise:
    - Leg press
    - Bench press
    - Weighted lunges
    - Shoulder press
    - Bicep curls
    - Triceps extensions using free weights
3. Feel great about your bod.

Doing HIRT twice a week is enough to reap its benefits, which are many. On top of targeting muscle, improving metabolism, and supporting bone density, the full-body workout is particularly good for women because it strengthens the muscle groups that can help us avoid common issues like knee, neck, and back pain.

It's important to make sure you're using weights so heavy that you can only perform *six to eight reps per set*. And if you're new to lifting, it's a good idea to watch videos online to learn proper technique—and to get a feel for a weight load that's appropriate. (Hot tip: At the end of the chapter, I've shared links to a few helpful resources, including a YouTube channel where you can search each exercise in the HIRT workout.) In general, women are usually weaker in the upper body, which means you'll use lighter weights for things like bicep curls and triceps extensions than you would for weighted lunges. You'll know you're ready to increase weight when you can do eight reps in every set, no problem.

Abbie admits doing HIRT at home can be tricky if you don't have dumbbells. And even if you do, they may not be heavy enough, so working out at a gym may be the best option. But the workout is flexible in that you can adjust for whatever you have at your disposal—if you have lighter weights at home, for example, consider shortening the rest times to make it higher intensity. If you don't have equipment for a leg press, like me, you can hold dumbbells on your shoulders to do a weighted squat instead.

There are plenty of other strength workouts to choose from, whether you find free programs online, sign up for structured programs such as the ECFIT Strength Series that Stacy created with a long-time strength coach specifically for women, or subscribe to apps (Nike Training Club is excellent, free, and provides tips on proper technique as you exercise).

Whatever you choose, lifting heavy is what counts. So do our nutritional choices. Stacy had already told me that you can't build muscle without an abundance of nutrition around exercise, and she pointed to Abbie's research as proof.

That's because Abbie and her team have shown that having a pre-workout snack with protein is most effective for women, contrary to the common belief that a post-workout snack with carbs is most important. When women consumed 90 calories of protein powder from a shake versus 90 calories of carbohydrates before exercising, the protein snack helped women burn more calories and fat after exercise.

You may need a post-workout snack, she says, if you have a particularly long and strenuous session. Otherwise, you can usually wait for your next meal. "All I would say is never go into exercise fasted," Abbie says. A good rule of thumb: "If you haven't eaten for three hours, you should have something."

Though you can get protein from whole foods like beans, Greek yogurt, eggs, and meat, the body will absorb a protein mixed with liquid much faster. The kind Abbie recommends is whey protein isolate, the highest-quality protein powder because the fat and lactose are filtered out. She prefers whey over plant-based and collagen proteins because the latter two are incomplete proteins that don't have enough leucine, which stimulates muscle. She wishes more women knew that to get enough protein from a plant protein, you must usually double or triple the serving size and ingest massive amounts of carbohydrate as a result. "With a whey protein, it's much easier to get 25 grams of protein," she says.

And getting enough protein as a woman is imperative. Baseline recommendations say women should get about 1.6 grams of protein per kilogram of body weight and even more if you're an aging woman interested in building muscle. At the bare minimum, we need about 80 to 90 grams of protein a day.

When she told me she's about 135 pounds and consumes 180 grams of protein a day, I was floored. I'd been tracking my protein intake for a week and was falling at least 30 grams short of the 100 grams a day she recommended for my 118-pound self. (Curious to know how much you're getting? The free protein calculator I used is also listed at the end of the chapter.)

To boost my intake, I decided to follow the experts' lead and ingest some protein powder bright and early. Stacy drinks a cold-brew coffee mixed with milk and a scoop of unflavored protein powder before her early-morning workouts.

Similarly, Abbie blends a shake with vanilla protein powder, coffee, ice, spinach, and berries to drink before working out or while she's getting her kids' breakfast ready.

After a bit of experimenting, I've landed on my ideal mix. First, I heat a cup of cow's milk in the microwave. Next, I stir a scoop of chocolate-flavored protein powder in, then use a frother to dissolve any remaining chunks and foam everything up. Last, I pour the protein blend over about a cup of coffee in my big travel mug. It's DELISH—think mocha vibes—and easy to drink while I eat my breakfast. It's also a simple way to make sure I'm adding a solid dose of protein to my diet. The rest of the day I just try to eat a bit more protein at every meal, which isn't hard but adds up quickly.

The protein content in seven common foods, courtesy of Today's Dietitian

FOOD	SERVING SIZE	CALORIES	PROTEIN (g)
Chicken, skinless	3 oz	141	28
Large egg	1 egg	71	6
Salmon	3 oz	155	22
Black beans	½ cup	114	8
Peanut butter	1 tbsp	188	7
Greek yogurt	6 oz	100	18
Milk, skim	1 cup	86	8

Now, before we move on to one last supplement to consider, I'm curious: Did you notice I mentioned *cow's* milk? And did it shake you to your core?

I ask because, like so many of my friends, prior to speaking with Abbie I'd been using oat or almond milk in my coffee and recipes. I don't really know why, other than I'd fallen for the hype about alternative milks, somehow thinking they were better for me than regular milk.

If you've been thinking that way too, Abbie has a message: Switch back to cow's milk. Now. Like, immediately. And if you're lactose intolerant, she recommends trying Fairlife or a2 milk to get similar, high-quality nutrition.

"I feel like milk got such a bad rap because it's got a lot of calories and it fills you up," Abbie says. "It doesn't mean you have to drink tons of it, but a 6-ounce glass of skim milk can have 8 to 10 grams of protein, plus it also provides calcium and vitamin D." It also has more electrolytes than processed milks, which means that mixing it with a bit of protein powder after a workout is an excellent way to rehydrate and recover faster.

She sold me. I haven't bought another kind of milk since. Not only do I like the taste, but it feels good knowing I'm supporting my muscle and bone health while I'm sipping a latte.

But getting more protein, be it from a latte, food, or powder, isn't the only way to support muscle health. Amino acids are the building blocks of protein; nine of the twenty are deemed essential amino acids (EAAs), yet the body can't produce them on its own. Because it's hard for us to get everything we need from food, Abbie says taking EAA supplements mixed with water before, during or after exercise is helpful for women, especially if you can't stomach a protein shake. They also come in handy when you need something to sustain you between meals.

EAA supplements promote muscle gain and recovery, but they also support everything from cognitive ability and metabolism to hormone regulation and cardiovascular health. The key is finding one with all nine EAAs, which isn't hard to spot with names like Dymatize All 9 Amino.

I struggle to drink enough water at the best of times, so mixing in a scoop of flavored powder sounded appealing. After speaking with Abbie, I jumped online to order one of the EAA supplements she'd recommended, a berry-flavored Amino Complex by Thorne Research. When it arrived—love at first sip, by the way—I felt ready to implement everything I'd learned.

I had the info! The workout strategy! The supplements, or as my husband jokingly called them when he opened our cupboard, "an array of potions and tinctures"! And thanks to a home scale that measures weight, muscle mass, and body fat, I also had baseline estimates to help gauge my results.

First, a pro tip: If you're serious about getting a precise body composition measurement, consider paying for a Bod Pod test (search "Bod Pod near me" online to find a location). The test is fast, non-invasive, offered at gyms and other organizations across North America, and, most importantly, much more accurate than a home scale or caliper test. I learned this years ago when writing about the various ways you can measure body composition—and was reminded of it again when writing this chapter. Not to bore you with numbers, but the two Bod Pod tests I had, the first one before I started my new fitness routine and the second many months into it, assessed my body fat much lower than my home scale and my muscle mass much higher. Both methods showed I was trending in the right direction, though, and knowing I was propelling myself toward my goal gave me an encouraging boost.

To be clear, my goal was not to lose weight. It was to get stronger, healthier, fitter—things we can all aspire to. I'll share my start and end numbers from my home scale below, but please keep in mind (a) results will vary because we are all gloriously different, and (b) I'm not a researcher, expert, or dietitian. I'm just a girl, standing in front of a bunch of girls, asking them to speak with their doctors before making changes to their wellness routines.

Cool? Great.

Here's a glimpse of how it went down when I put everything into action.

Day 1
Weight: 118 lbs
Muscle mass: 73.5% or 86.7 lbs
Mood: Excited to start a new routine

Started my day with my usual bowl of oatmeal and a yummy protein coffee, ate lunch, and then ate a bowl of plain Greek yogurt before tackling a Peloton strength class at 2:30 p.m. It had been three hours since my lunch and I am nothing if not a rule follower. Instead of reaching for my usual 10-pound and 15-pound weights for my arm and leg exercises, I grabbed 15s and 20s. I struggled to get some moves done, like squats and overhead presses, but I managed and felt strong. Ten minutes after the workout, I congratulated myself with a homemade granola bar, complete with 8 grams of protein, some carbs and, if you must know, a hefty dose of M&Ms.

Day 2
Mood: Does being sore in muscles you didn't know you had count as a mood?

Even though I'd planned to try Abbie's HIIT workout on my bike, I listened to my body and took it easy. I ate a granola bar before going for a 45-minute walk to get some fresh air. Soon after I got back home, my husband walked in the door carrying two new 30-pound weights for his own workouts. He'd seen me using his 20s the day before and thought, "I need to up my game. And, damn, my wife is hot!" I may be paraphrasing. Either way, as of day 2, we were *both* lifting heavier shit.

Day 3
Mood: Ready for a sweaty HIIT workout

Started my day with protein coffee—obsessed!—and ate my usual meals. Instead of having a pre-workout granola bar, I mixed the EAA blend into a big water bottle and drank about half before jumping onto the bike at 3 p.m. Tackled Abbie's HIIT routine, alternating between one minute of all-out effort and one minute of rest. Felt like puking after interval No. 4. Scaled back a bit and felt better around interval No. 7. Managed to finish all ten intervals, sipped my EAAs afterward and floated on a post-workout high for the rest of the day. Note to self: Go a little easier on the intervals next time.

Day 13

Mood: Oozing bad-ass, superwoman vibes

I bought a pair of black gloves for weight training because gripping heavier weights was hurting my palms. Wore them for a HIRT session today and they helped. Bonus: I felt so sexy—like '80s Madonna in her gloves—that I was dancing around to my music during the rest periods. I'm loving HIRT and pushing myself to lift heavier all the time, no matter the workout. Hubby is not impressed I'm already stealing his 30-pound weights for my lunges.

Day 21

Mood: Feeling well-rested and less sore

I realized I'm sleeping much better. My legs used to ache at night—that pain is gone! huzzah!—and I'm falling asleep easier, too. I'm not sure it's 100 percent thanks to the EAAs I'm drinking every day, but I have a hunch they're helping. Also, my HIIT workouts don't make me nauseous anymore. Small victories, my friends.

Fast forward to today: Day 120

Weight: 118 lbs

Muscle mass: 75.2% or 88.7 lbs

Mood: Look at me go! Building muscle! Feeling good!

Every day, I genuinely look forward to taking my two supplements, and I usually get two HIIT and two HIRT workouts in per week. Altogether, the four sessions amount to an hour-and-a-half of exercise a week. I used to put that time into one workout! Sometimes I don't get all the workouts done or I swap one out for a Peloton class or long walk because I love those activities. And I'm so happy with the results.

Though I weigh the same as when I started, I've added two pounds of muscle, which means I've lost some body fat. That's a trend I want to maintain, so I'll be sticking with this routine. It's not just the numbers that are motivating me. I *feel* better. I'm able lift my kids with less effort and have more energy to get me through the day. Shorter workouts also mean I feel less stress about fitting them in. And as for brain fog, has it improved?

Hmm. What was the question again?

Kidding! I don't notice a difference in my mental prowess, but I do notice I have better definition in my arm muscles and a plumper tush. *Ooh la la.*

The biggest takeaway for me has been this: I've finally embraced the idea that exercise doesn't have to be hours long to be effective. Exercising smart trumps exercising a lot, every time. And having that knowledge is so liberating.

When you give this fitness strategy a shot, I hope you feel the same way. And as you start out, please don't think you have to try everything at once. Make one change, and then maybe try another.

Regardless of where you're at on your fitness journey, it's never too late to switch things up. "Women are so hard on themselves, but tomorrow's a new day," as Abbie told me. "No matter what you've done before, you can build muscle and improve your bone mineral density. The body adapts to what you do to it, and I think that's exciting."

As do I. You can do this, ladies! We can do this!

And here's the cheat sheet to help keep us on track.

THE CHEAT SHEET

- If you do only one thing, lift weights two to three times per week. Strength training is critical for maintaining muscle, especially as we age.
- Challenge yourself to lift heavy. You will not bulk up, but you will get stronger.
- Aim for two interval training workouts per week. Keep them short and intense! You'll reap all the benefits of cardio without sacrificing hours of your life.
- Do any activity or movement that brings you joy.
- Do not exercise fasted. If you haven't eaten within three hours, eat or drink a pre-workout snack with protein. And if you have a long and strenuous session, have a post-workout snack with protein, too.
- Stop skipping meals. Getting nutrition throughout the day not only means you'll have more energy to tackle high-quality workouts, but you'll avoid the long-term effects of intermittent fasting, like muscle loss and a slower metabolism.
- If you're not lactose intolerant, consume cow's milk. Compared to processed options like oat and almond, cow's milk has much more protein and nutritional value. Milk, indeed, does a body good.
- Consider incorporating whey protein isolate powder and essential amino acids into your daily routine. They're versatile, taste good and will help you meet your protein needs.

Four Helpful Links

- A YouTube channel where you can search specific exercises and watch video demos: www.youtube.com/c/MyTrainingApp

- A free recipe calculator to help you figure out how much protein you're getting: www.myfitnesspal.com/recipe/calculator
- A visual guide to protein serving sizes: www.thekitchn.com/a-visual-guide-to-protein-serving-sizes-243496
- A Stacy Sims–recommended site that sells high-quality whey protein isolate powders and ships to many countries: canadianprotein.com/

CHAPTER TWO

Get the Best Skin of Your Life

Yes, in Your Forties

THIS MAY NOT BE THE CHAPTER YOU'RE EXPECTING TO READ.

I'm telling you now so you understand (a) where I'm coming from and (b) what you *can* expect. As for the latter, this chapter is packed with tips on how to care for your skin using effective, accessible products. Following them will help reverse any damage you may have done when you were young, improve your skin's appearance and set your skin up for long-term health.

As for where I'm coming from, I can sum it up in one word: defiance.

That's because every place I look, I see solutions to "fix" my aging face. I know you see them, too, with all the magazine ads and Instagram posts and faces that look like they've been airbrushed. Got wrinkles? Get Botox. Sunken cheeks? Try dermal filler. Thin lips? There are injections for that.

Despite me having all those imperfections—and some vertical lines above my top lip that deepen every year—I refuse to believe that an aging face is unattractive or unworthy. The most perfect face in the world to me is my mother's, complete with the lines that reflect her laughter, her experiences, her love. I want that type of face when I'm older. I want to *see* those kinds of faces as I get older.

I'm so over the ridiculous idea that we must erase and hide our age that I once posted about it on Instagram, saying: "I want to celebrate our aging faces—wrinkles, fine lines, spots, and all." I was curious to hear how other women felt, so I asked them to share their thoughts.

And their posts were fantastic.

Take, for example, my friend Nadia Hrkac, who's ten years older than me and has always inspired my approach to aging. Here's what she wrote: "Never had anything done as I truly believe in aging gracefully and naturally. Not against it but want to embrace looking the way nature intended without the pressure of preserving the way we looked at a certain age. Being your true, authentic self is liberating."

Yes, Nadia. Hell yes. *That's* an idea I can get behind.

Because here's how I see it. We've come a long, long way in body positivity. We now celebrate all sizes and shapes, all body types and abilities. But we've yet to extend that self-love to the face. Why? Just as I hope my daughter Marlowe grows up feeling confident about the shape and size of her body, I hope she grows up knowing she doesn't have to do anything to her face.

For her sake and my own, I'm striving to embrace the skin I have.

Is it always easy? Not at all. As women, we are incredibly hard on ourselves. And I have not escaped that gene. I get annoyed when I see a new line dig in above my upper lip or a wrinkle settle into my forehead. But every day, I try to accept the woman I see in the mirror—and to pursue a more realistic goal than society would have me chase.

Here's what I *am* after as a woman in my forties: dewy, clear skin that looks as healthy as possible for my age now, through midlife and beyond. Celebrity facialist Joanna Czech nailed it for me when she told *InStyle* magazine in November 2021, "Aging is a privilege. Glowing skin with lines can be super sexy."

Yes, Joanna. Hell yes. *That's* a skin philosophy I can get behind.

No matter your approach to dealing with your skin, I'm here for it. I respect every woman's choice, as I hope others respect mine. You do you. I'll do me. Let's all just make sure we're doing everything we can daily to nourish and protect our skin.

To find out how, I turned to board-certified dermatologist Dr. Tina Alster, the founding director of the Washington Institute of Dermatologic Laser Surgery and a clinical professor of dermatology at Georgetown University. She wrote the first textbook on cosmetic laser surgery and has served as a consultant to skincare companies such as Lancôme and La Mer.

I'd contacted Tina because not only is she an award-winning expert in her field but, with an office two blocks from the White House, she sees a lot of patients like you and me: women who have little time for self-care but big wants for great skin.

When we connected on WhatsApp one evening, she told me why so many of us see visible signs of aging as we enter midlife.

"It's when the sins of your past catch up with you," Tina says.

Even if women take good care of their skin as they get older, chances are they paid little attention to sun protection when they were young. And while chronological aging and genetics are certainly factors in how we age, she said sun damage is what *really* ages our skin.

Ugh. I felt like she was staring into my soul. Or at the discoloration on my chest.

That's where I used to get a sunburn at least once a summer as a teenager. As an adult, I didn't fare much better. I spent two decades running and hiking outdoors without wearing sunscreen or a hat. And my overall skincare routine was haphazard at best. In short, I had not done my skin any favors.

Tina said her patients often see the signs of sun damage—fine lines, sunspots, and blotchiness—as early as their thirties and definitely by the time they're in their forties.

I can relate. My pigmentation, wrinkles, and uneven skin tone were getting more pronounced as I moved toward my forties. If that's what you've been noticing on your skin, too, don't fret.

"Sort of like it's never too late to stop smoking, it's never too late to start protecting your skin," Tina assured me. "It becomes your new starting point, but you have to dial back the damage."

I asked Tina how we can do that. Her advice was simple: Protect during the day. Repair at night.

To protect skin during the day, Tina recommends sun protection. But any old sunscreen won't do. It *must* be mineral sunblock.

"It's not because I'm natural schmatural," she said, "it's because chemical sunblocks actually absorb the heat from the sun and can irritate the skin. Mineral sunblocks reflect the sun and reduce the inflammation and heat that you can get from being outside."

If you have time and money to incorporate another product in your morning routine, she suggests layering a vitamin C serum or lotion underneath the sunblock. Antioxidants such as vitamin C add a second layer of protection from the sun and help prevent both wrinkles and sagging.

Another nice-to-have? Eye cream applied after your vitamin C product and before your sunblock.

"I do 1, 2, 3," she said. "After washing, put the active ingredient on, put your eye cream on, put your sunblock on. Period."

As for the second pillar in Tina's essential skincare program, repairing the skin at night depends on her patients' concerns. But if you're like me—a woman who's showing visible signs of aging and, yes, has some concerns about it—there's one skincare ingredient you need in your life, if you're not pregnant or breastfeeding.

Ladies, meet vitamin A, your new best friend.

Wait, you've already met. If you flip through magazines or watch talk shows or occasionally wander through Sephora, you know about vitamin A and its many derivatives, called retinoids.

On the weaker end of the retinoid scale, you have retinyl esters such as retinyl palmitate and retinyl acetate. As you move up its food chain in strength, Tina explained, you find retinol. The strongest retinoid is retinoic acid, a prescription-strength form of vitamin A commonly known as Retin-A.

Retinoids are the gold-standard ingredient for good reason. They've been scientifically proven to increase cell turnover, fade sunspots, treat acne, lessen fine lines and wrinkles, and promote collagen production. Considering collagen production starts to decline sometime in our twenties or thirties, any help we can get in maintaining our skin's plump, supple glow is a good thing.

Even if you're familiar with retinoids, there's something you may not know: You don't need to use the strongest retinoid to reap vitamin A's benefits. Prescription-strength retinoids such as Retin-A may give you results faster, but they're often too irritating for women to handle.

As I've found out after years of experimenting with prescription-strength gels and over-the-counter creams, most retinoids are too strong for me. They leave my skin peeling and red, even if I apply them only one or two nights a week. But given everything I'd read and heard—and even been prescribed—I mistakenly believed strong meant best. I'm not alone.

"I think most dermatologists say, 'You have to be using a retinoic acid,' but most of my patients have never been able to use retinoic acid or Retin-A every night without irritation," Tina said. "Some only use it twice a week, but it still irritates their skin. Why even have it on your shelf?"

A far better option is applying a weaker retinoid every night that won't irritate your skin. For that reason, Tina herself uses retinol instead of retinoic acid. Consistently applying a lesser-strength retinoid will yield the magical results vitamin A is known for. It just might take more time.

No matter your skin color, Tina's advice is the same: Protect during the day and repair at night. If you have melanated skin and struggle with hyper-pigmentation or melasma, then she'd recommend adding one more product at night to enhance the repair process—topical tranexamic acid. And if you're in the market for one, Tina developed a serum called Advanced TX Lightening Gel Elixir to lighten and correct skin discoloration. (She created a whole line of derm-quality skincare products. You can find them at theamethod.com.)

I asked Tina if women need a special moisturizer or night cream to round out the nighttime routine or in the morning, for that matter. Only if your skin is dry, she said. Depending on where you live, the condition of your skin, and how it reacts to the active ingredients you're using, you may not need one at all. But if, like me, you live in a dry city and your skin is a scaly mess without moisturizer, add it to your routine.

Tina doesn't need moisturizer, so her process is even shorter at nighttime than in the morning. She washes her face, then applies retinol and eye cream. That's it! So easy! As she said, "You can always add things later, like a neck, elbow, or foot cream, but not before you put the good stuff on."

I know the good stuff works because, a handful of months before my conversation with her, I received similar advice from a facialist who's based in my hometown.

When I visited Stacey Irvine for the first time in April 2021, I was expecting a relaxing facial and maybe a few tips. But an education on the subtleties of skincare? Now that was a surprise.

I found Stacey as we find most things these days: on Instagram. A registered nurse specializing in functional medicine, she decided to pursue her passion and become a skin therapist. She is generous with her knowledge, sharing product advice, skincare tips, and much more on social media (check her out at @staceyirvineskin). Most importantly, she has the healthiest skin I'd ever seen. Her bright, dewy, thirty-something skin radiates in every post, every story.

I yearned for that kind of skin.

Reading Stacey's approach online convinced me she was the facialist I needed. In her words, "I simply adore helping humans to restore the vibrancy and glow of their skin while helping them to remember their most whole and authentic self."

I was a human in need of vibrant and glowing skin. Remembering my whole and authentic self, I thought, would be a bonus.

For the first half hour of my session at her clinic in Calgary, Alberta, we talked about every skincare product I'd been using, namely the Costco-brand face wipes I'd been using to take my makeup off at night, a facial scrub I'd bought at Sephora on a whim, a handful of serums lining my shelves, some sheet masks I grabbed at the drugstore, the strong retinoic acid a dermatologist had prescribed in passing when I mentioned my fine lines, and a moisturizer/sunscreen blend I wore under my makeup.

I could have saved us both time and just said, "I have no idea what I'm doing. Please help."

When she asked about my concerns, my number-one was, obviously, aging and how to do it well. I added that my skin had looked blotchy, dull, and irritated for many months. What was I doing wrong?

Plenty. And it all came down to my skin barrier function.

"The skin barrier is like a brick wall. It's designed to prevent things from coming into the skin and to help prevent things from leaving the skin, in particular transepidermal water loss," she said. "When people have different manifestations of skin conditions, whether it's pigmentation or acne or aging, at the end of the day it doesn't even matter what their skin type is. What I really care about is the health of the skin barrier. And my only job is to figure out how to help nourish that."

In my case, my brick wall was shoddy. And the main culprit was those Kirkland face wipes, which were stripping my skin of its natural oils. But it's not just the face wipes that are problematic. Stacey says cleansers with emulsifiers, which are designed to keep oil and water from separating and give products longer shelf lives, are hard on skin.

"People will spend loads of money on serums and moisturizers but have their cleanser wrong. That's the first step of your program, so if you're starting it by creating a deficiency in the skin, the products that follow it won't work as well."

That's why, to help keep a youthful glow, it's smart to use a gentle face cleanser. "When you put an emulsifying face wash on your skin, the product will look for the oil in your skin to be able to mix it with the water," she said, "and then you'll wash it down the drain. The moment you use a frothy cleanser or anything with an emulsifier, you're unintentionally aging yourself."

Spotting emulsifiers in a product's ingredient list is complicated, so Stacey tells her clients that if a cleanser gets frothy or foamy as you wash your face, it likely has emulsifying agents. Another telltale sign? Your skin feels tight or dry after washing.

A Facialist's Go-To Drink

Stacey Irvine, a registered nurse–turned–skin therapist who refers to herself as a "skin nerd," rarely drinks wine because "alcohol is really hard on skin." But she loves a good margarita.

Tequila is the easiest alcohol on skin, she says, because it has less sugar than wine and beer. Less sugar means less glycation, a process that hardens collagen and makes skin less supple.

To make her go-to margarita, you'll need:

1 oz tequila
½ oz Grand Marnier
1 full, freshly squeezed lime
Soda water
Lots of ice

Mix the first three ingredients in a shaker. Pour into a glass with a salted rim and top with soda water. Stir. Enjoy.

Much like a foaming cleanser, my face wipes were stripping essential oils from my skin, so she suggested I switch to a milk cleanser. And instead of washing my face with hot water, as I usually do because I'm always cold, she made me promise to use cold water. "Hot water is so drying and inflammatory," she explained.

Most importantly, she asked me to stop using every scrub, toner, mask, and serum that I'd been experimenting with and stick to the basic steps: wash, moisturize, protect.

For the latter two steps, Stacey suggested I ditch my moisturizer/sunscreen combo because two-in-one products that promise to moisturize *and* protect tend to fall short in both regards. "Those are two different products you should not blend because they have significant roles to play on the skin," she said. "Your moisturizer should be like skin food and your SPF should be SPF."

Good moisturizers have skin-boosting ingredients like ceramides and vitamins that are meant to be absorbed by the skin. SPF, on the other hand, should not be absorbed. That's why she, too, recommends using mineral sunblock with titanium dioxide and zinc oxide, the two minerals most effective at blocking UVA and UVB rays.

Aside from protecting skin from the sun, mineral sunblock provides an unexpected aesthetic bonus. "When I'm trying to make my skin look really dewy and glowy, I use my mineral sunblock," said Stacey, adding that her product of choice is Eclipse SPF 50+ by iS Clinical, a professional skincare brand. "It gives the skin a luminosity."

After the most informative facial I'd ever had, I left Stacey's clinic with two new products I needed to follow her advice: cleansing milk called Lait E.V. by Biologique Recherche, a French skincare brand, and a retinyl palmitate moisturizer called Skin EssentiA by Environ, a brand that believes "skin has a life, and that vitamin A is the 'oxygen' it needs to look beautiful and healthy."

A few weeks later—because a girl can only drop so much money at one appointment, am I right?—I bought the iS Clinical mineral sunblock, too.

Compared to my Costco facial wipes and Neutrogena SPF moisturizer, my new products cost a *lot* more. I was hoping they'd be worth it, especially since I'd invested in a moisturizer that could work double duty, with application both day and night. Though retinoids are typically only meant for nighttime use, Environ recommends using its moisturizer before bed *and* in the morning. And because retinoids make skin more sensitive to UV rays, applying sunblock on top would be critical.

Here's what happened when I implemented a minimal skincare routine:

Day 1

Jumped out of bed excited to wash my face. (Is that weird?) Took my time rubbing the Biologique Recherche milk cleanser into my skin and, because Stacey mentioned the product is filled with things that do the skin good, let it sit on my skin while I brushed my teeth. Kept the cold water running (eeks) and wet a soft microfiber facial cloth—yet another Stacey suggestion—then used it to gently wipe the cleanser from my face. Surprise #1: cold water feels incredible! And refreshing! I'm more awake! Surprise #2: My skin immediately feels less tight and more supple. It's like the cleanser hydrated my skin before I'd even applied any other products. Next, I applied two pumps of Environ's Vita-Antioxidant AVST Moisturiser 2; the company offers a five-step, graduated system with increasing levels of retinyl palmitate, and since I had some experience using retinol, I started at level two. I followed that up with some drugstore-brand eye cream I already owned and slathered mineral sunblock on my face and the backs of my hands. My skin looked so dewy, and makeup application was a breeze.

Final thought: Adding a couple of products to my morning routine adds some time, but I don't mind. It feels good knowing I'm on the right skin track.

Night 1

Had a long day and just wanted to crawl into bed. Using a facial wipe was tempting, but I reached for the milk cleanser and microfiber cloth and repeated the same washing process. I followed that up with the Environ moisturizer and my eye cream and called it a day.

Final thought: The nighttime routine is so quick and simple. Love it!

Week 3

My skin is already looking much better! It's visibly plumper, not to mention less red and irritated. Nixing the facial wipes is obviously helping, as is using a retinoid that's mild enough for my skin to handle (see ya, redness and flaking). My skin feels stronger and more elastic. Is my brick wall firming up? I believe so. And I've even started to look forward to washing my face with cold water. Who knew it was so refreshing? I don't notice a difference in my wrinkles yet—I use one line that's above my upper lip on the right side of my face as a barometer—but knowing my skin is already healthier and plumper gives me hope.

Final thought: I can't believe how much my skin has improved in less than a month. For the first time in my life, I feel like glowing skin is in reach.

Month 3

I've been following my new routine religiously, protecting skin during the day and repairing it at night. I haven't exfoliated once, applied a face mask, or used any of the random products that are currently gathering dust in my bathroom. And the results are even better than before! My crow's feet have softened, my face is smoother, and my sunspots have all but disappeared, leaving my skin tone even and clear. I AM A HAPPY WOMAN. For real. Like, that line above my upper lip? It's plumped up somehow; so, while I can still see a faint indentation, it's not as noticeable.

Final thought: Quality skincare = magic.

Month 9

Time to kick things up a notch! Now that I'm comfortable with my new routine and my finances have recovered from that initial spend on skincare, I invested in a vitamin C serum to use underneath my moisturizer and sunblock. My choice? The Super Serum Advance + by iS Clinical, touted as being "amazing for brightening and protecting skin, and also at helping to even skin tone and reduce the appearance of dark spots." Time will tell.

Final thought: On initial application, the serum feels watery and tacky. But it works well under the products layered on top. Do your thing, vitamin C!

Month 12

Well, can't say I'm in love with the vitamin C serum. I don't notice a difference in my skin, but the eternal optimist in me must believe it's been working on a deeper level, and that, uh, good stuff will ensue? I don't know. I DO know that I'm willing to give another vitamin C product a try. And as luck would have it, I recently watched every second of Phoebe Dynevor's video for *Vogue*, in which she shares her skincare and beauty secrets. (Have you seen season one of "Bridgerton"? Her skin is *flawless.*) She swears by Sunday Riley's C.E.O. 15% Vitamin C Brightening Serum, so that's what I just started using. Hopes are high, my friends.

Final thought: I've been using this lotion for a month and, wow, it's true love. I much prefer this consistency—it's thicker than the iS Clinical serum, hydrating, and soaks in immediately. It's not sticky and plays well with everything I put on top of it. And in just four weeks, I can tell my skin is brighter, clearer, and glowier than usual. Girls, I think I've made it. I have reached my version of skin nirvana.

You'll note, however, that my nirvana does not include the consumption of collagen powder.

In case you missed it, collagen supplements have been all the rage for a while.

Collagen supplements are made of peptides, which are amino acids the body can easily absorb. And ingesting them regularly is supposed to minimize fine lines and wrinkles, repair sun damage, increase skin hydration, improve bone density, and more.

Enticing stuff, indeed.

The idea of mixing a flavorless collagen powder into my coffee to give me all those benefits sounded nifty, so I gave it a try a few years ago. After using a marine-sourced collagen powder every day for more than two months, I didn't notice any changes. I reached out to Dr. Lisa Kellett, a board-certified dermatologist in Toronto, to get her thoughts. She wasn't surprised by my results, or lack thereof.

"There's no evidence-based medicine to support the use of these powders. And remember, if you're ingesting collagen powder, it goes into your bowel, so you're basically excreting it."

Great. I literally flushed $75 down the drain.

Lisa recommended I stick to wearing sun protection every day with a vitamin C serum underneath (yes, the antioxidant we just discussed) and a vitamin A product at night (yes, the retinoid we just discussed). "There's evidence to show those things *will* improve skin."

Three years have passed since then, but the science behind supplements hasn't evolved much. Nor have many opinions.

"I have no time for collagen powder," Tina told me during our chat. "You're far better off applying a cream with peptides directly on your skin than drinking peptides that need to find their way to the skin."

That's why, until science proves me otherwise, I'll be taking my coffee with milk and protein powder. Hold the collagen.

And in case you're wondering, just like with supplements, there's no one food that will give you great skin. According to Vivien Fam, who was a dietitian and clinical research scientist at Integrative Skin Science and Research in Sacramento, California, before she passed away in 2023, eating a wide array of nutritious foods is our best option.

When we chatted via Google Meet one afternoon, Vivien told me she grew up in Malaysia with a mother who knew how powerful food could be in more ways than one. On top of feeding her family many good-for-you things, her mom would use ingredients like cucumber paste, puréed pumpkin, oatmeal, and honey to make homemade face masks.

Even with all her exposure to nutritious foods, Vivien says she didn't think about the connection between food and skin until she began studying nutrition at the University of New Hampshire years later. As she told me, "The idea of nutrition and skin health is relatively new, even now. Although skin is the largest organ, we're more aware of how nutrition affects our inner organs than what's on the outside."

Fam's research helped to change that. Despite the articles we've all read touting "The Best Foods to Eat for Your Skin," very few whole foods have been clinically researched. "I'm not saying that lists with those foods being good for skin are wrong, but those ideas came about because the foods are rich in certain vitamins—and there's a lot of research on how vitamins affect skin," she said. "What I'm talking about is how *food* affects skin, and there's a difference."

Whole foods contain vitamins, minerals, and nutrients that work together, so how a particular combination affects skin isn't clear. Vivien's own study is a good example. She hypothesized that postmenopausal women eating fresh or frozen nutrient-rich mangos would see improvement in wrinkles and overall skin health. Postmenopausal women are often used in skin studies, she said, because they don't have hormonal fluctuations confounding findings. And, unlike younger women, they have wrinkles that can be measured.

Four times a week for sixteen weeks, Vivien had one group of women eat half a cup of mangos and another group eat 1.5 cups. She expected the group eating more mangos would see the biggest improvements thanks to more vitamin C. That's not what happened. Their wrinkles worsened, while the group on the half-cup regimen saw an improvement. "We don't know why, but we speculate that the sugar from the mangos might have caused glycation and the increase in wrinkles."

That's why Vivien suggested women limit their sugar intake and consume colorful fruits and vegetables of all kinds, as well as nuts and legumes. In particular, and as she outlined in a published review on skin health and nutrition, nutrient-rich foods such as kale, tomatoes, almonds, melon, mangos, pomegranate, oranges, grapes, and soy can have beneficial effects on skin health, but more research is needed. She and her co-authors concluded that eating an abundance of plant-based foods is desirable, but overconsuming a single food or extract is not.

Moderation, it seems, is the key to glowing skin on many fronts—skincare, food, and even lifestyle. That's what my final interviewee about skincare highlighted when we spoke in the fall of 2021.

Dr. Diane Berson, a board-certified dermatologist based in New York City, had just left a skincare conference and was sitting in the back of a car, en route to the airport and then on to Chicago for an American Academy of Dermatology board of directors meeting. During our phone call, we covered skincare basics—she reiterated how essential vitamin A, vitamin C, and mineral sunblock are for aging women—but what struck me most was her answer to my last question, which was: Is there anything else you're passionate about sharing with women in midlife?

Start with a Skin Check

When you hit 40, it's time to see a dermatologist. But not for the reason you think. Every adult woman needs a head-to-toe skin cancer check, says board-certified dermatologist Dr. Diane Berson. "Skin cancer incidences have gone up and some skin cancers can be fatal. That's why everyone should see a dermatologist for a baseline skin cancer check."

Once you've got that done, she says, you can segue into discussing the fun stuff, like getting onto an effective skincare routine and exploring treatments to help address your concerns. But getting the check is paramount and, bonus, it's free in most places.

The American Academy of Dermatology has offered a free skin cancer screening program since 1985, its longest-standing public health program. Head to aad.org/public to find a skin cancer screening option near you. In Canada, ask your family doctor about getting referred to a dermatologist. Coverage varies by province, but skin checks are often free if you're referred.

"Don't feel like you have to do everything and be everything to everyone," she said without hesitation. "Make sure to take time for yourself because when you're happier, you look healthier. Of course, as a dermatologist I'd like to know you're using a very good skincare routine. But pay attention to your sleep, diet, hydration, exercise, and whatever you need to do to feel confident, whether it's running ten miles or taking a warm bath or having a glass of wine."

Self-care like that has always made me happy, but I'd never thought about how that feeling was translating to my face. It makes total sense, though. Now, whenever I pour a glass of rosé and hop in the bath, or go for a walk and listen to music, or even take time to read before bed, I remind myself I'm doing my mood *and* my skin good.

Most importantly, I've been keeping up with my minimal skincare routine. And the effects continue to astound me. My skin is better than ever—even better than in my twenties. Overall, the improvement in my skin has been so drastic that even my friends have noticed and asked what products I'm using. When I told them, they were surprised at how few there are in my daily routine.

Now that I'm far into this experiment, I've finally donated or tossed all the masks, scrubs, and toners I'd pushed to the back of my shelves. Not only do I have more room, but I have more money. Though my new skincare lineup is pricier per product, I need fewer because they're more effective.

As for my wrinkles? They're still there, albeit less noticeable—for now. I know my lines will grow and deepen with age. And I'm cool with that. I want to look healthy and vibrant for my age, be the sexy gal with glowing skin and lines. When I struggle to feel that way, as I'm sure I will, I'll remind myself of women like my friend Nadia who are living unapologetically as themselves. I'll keep choosing to love the woman I see in the mirror. And I'll feel confident knowing I'm taking exceptional care of my skin, day in and day out.

Here's the cheat sheet with some helpful reminders on how we can all do just that.

THE CHEAT SHEET

- Establish a simple at-home skincare routine that works for your skin. If your face is red and irritated, try scaling back on the number of products you're using. Stick to the few that protect skin during the day and repair it at night.
- If you apply only one product in the morning, make it a mineral sunblock with titanium dioxide and zinc oxide.
- To ramp up your morning routine, apply a vitamin C serum and an eye cream underneath your sunblock.
- If you apply only one product at night, make it a vitamin A–derived retinoid. Not everyone can handle full-strength

retinoic acid, so don't be afraid to try products with milder derivatives such as retinol or retinyl palmitate.

- Use a gentle, non-foaming face wash to cleanse morning and night. While you're at it, use cold water instead of hot water to reduce dryness and inflammation.
- Apply moisturizer if your skin is dry. In the morning, apply it after your serum and eye cream but before sunblock. At night, you can apply moisturizer before or after a retinoid product, depending on the consistency of both. The general rule is to apply products from thinnest/lightest to thickest/heaviest.
- Limit your sugar intake and eat all kinds of nutritious foods. Plant-based foods seem to be especially good for the skin.
- Take time for the activities you love. When you're happier, you look healthier.
- If you haven't yet by the time you turn 40, see a dermatologist to get a full-body skin cancer check.
- Follow pro-aging advocates on social media. Women like Paulina Porizkova and Denise Boomkens share inspiring posts about aging that are good for the soul. They do mine good, anyway!

CHAPTER THREE

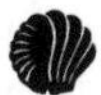

Put Your Best Face Forward

Over the pandemic, I developed a new pastime: studying Sutton Foster's face. Sutton was the lead actress on "Younger," an addictive TV show starring Hilary Duff, Debi Mazar, and other babes that I binge-watched at night. The show kicks off with Sutton struggling to find work as a 40-something. The solution? A makeover that helps her pass for a girl in her mid-twenties and land an entry-level job at a publishing house. As a 40-something woman who's interested in looking as youthful and vibrant as possible, I loved watching Sutton fool her coworkers.

I was also desperate to learn her makeup secrets.

Because do you know which other face I was busy evaluating during the pandemic?

My own.

Nearly every workday from home, I'd end up in a virtual meeting. Sure, I *looked* at the other participants—what am I, a monster?—but I would inevitably be drawn to the square with my own mug and gaze into my tired, puffy eyes, wondering if any makeup tricks could brighten my face.

I mean, forget about makeup tricks. I just needed to know how to do my makeup, plain and simple. I'd been following the same routine since having a MAC Cosmetics lesson when I was

16. I was pretty sure things had changed since then—for both makeup *and* my face—so I decided to do something about it.

Enter Eldo Ray Estes, the Emmy-winning makeup artist known for his work on "Younger," "Orange Is the New Black," and "A Simple Favor," among other shows and films. His clients include Sharon Stone, Annette Bening, Debi Mazar, and Judith Light. All lovely, mature faces.

After watching the "Younger" series finale in 2021, I reached out to see if Eldo would be willing to share his advice for women in their forties. The New York–based celebrity makeup artist kindly agreed to divulge his secrets. Within the first few minutes of our chat one Sunday morning, he confirmed my hunch: Beauty routines must evolve with age. "If any woman is doing the same makeup she was doing at 18 when she's 40, she needs to seriously rethink it," he said.

I am that woman! I am rethinking!

If you are too, Eldo has some suggestions.

Eldo Ray Estes's Product Recommendations

Here are a few products he loves to use on clients, many of whom are older:

1. Armani Beauty's **Luminous Silk Foundation**: "It's a great product and it comes in about 40 different shades."
2. Shiseido's **Oil-Control Blotting Paper**: "I keep them in my bag because I use them all the time."
3. Christian Dior's eyeshadow palette in **Nude Dress**: "I'm using it on everybody right now."
4. Blinc's **Original Tubing Mascara**: "It kind of coats the lash with a little tube of plastic and it doesn't run."
5. Anastasia's **Brow Wiz** or Kevyn Aucoin's **Precision Brow Pencil**: "They're both hard and skinny, so you can get delicate, hair-like strokes."

First, he said, consider buying a foundation that doesn't need to be powdered. "Powder is not a good thing after a certain age," he said. "When you keep powdering your face, it changes your makeup and settles into fine lines and wrinkles." If oil strikes—and let's be real, it's impossible to avoid—Eldo uses blotting papers. Wondering what to use exactly? See the box with his product recommendations.

Second, Eldo says older women should stop applying eye makeup—eyeliner, mascara, and eyeshadow—under their eyes. Turns out that was one of the ways he kept Sutton looking so fresh. "On 'Younger,' Sutton never, ever, ever had eyeliner underneath her eyes. We didn't even use mascara on the bottom." Why so bare? "You always want to keep the focus up. It scares women to leave the undereye clean, but trust me. It makes a big difference."

Last, and to help keep the focus up, he suggests two more strategies: Define your brows every day because "brows give the face a structure," and apply eyeliner only from the outside corner to the middle of the upper lid. "Using a pencil, start the line on the outside and let it disappear by the time you hit the arch," he said, adding that it's almost like creating a little wedge. "Then smudge it out using a powder liner brush and an eyeshadow that's maybe a shade lighter than the pencil. It will give you the illusion of a wing and lift the corners of your eyes." Bonus: Using eyeshadow to fade the line out not only softens the look but sets the pencil and protects it from running.

After our call—and buoyed by the idea that change is good—I put Eldo's tips into action. One of the biggest changes I've focused on is defining my brows. And I *need* to focus because I'm terrible at it. See, my brows are thin, oh so thin. But they were once thick, oh so thick. My mom took me for electrolysis when I was a teen to save me from an unfortunate unibrow situation. After that was dealt with, we should have stopped. It was the '90s, though, and thin brows were hot, so I kept going for appointments. Did you know electrolysis uses electricity to zap individual hairs at the root and remove them permanently? My brows are the proof it works. Nearly thirty years have passed, and I wish I still had 90 percent of the hair we zapped.

Alas, I can't do anything about it now. For years, I'd go for the occasional brow appointment to get them trimmed but put zero effort into filling them. Eldo encouraged me to give it a go. So, I bought one of the pencils he recommended, and every day I draw on thin hairs, brush my brows up, and then hold them in place with a clear brow gel. I'm getting better—and I see the difference full brows make to my face.

In case you're wondering, yes, I've considered having them micro-bladed. But I've seen some great micro-bladed brows and some . . . not so great. And the idea of having not-so-great brows semi-permanently tattooed on my face scares me. I already have a faded tattoo of a shooting star on my right butt cheek that I could live without. Having botched brows on my face? I would never leave the house. Eldo dissuaded me from getting them tattooed, as well. "You need to be old school and learn how to draw your eyebrows on," he told me. "There's a little bit of work involved, but it's worth it."

To eliminate *some* of the work, I decided to finally try something my brow girl had been recommending for a few years: brow lamination or, as it's sometimes called, a brow lift. She described it to me as a perm for brows and promised it would make them look full, luscious, and well groomed. Considering my eyebrows are thin *and* unruly—how lucky am I?—I was into the idea of taming them while making them look fuller.

But I was also terrified. Would I like them? Would my husband?

Yes, I agree—it's only my opinion that matters. But my brows had stunned us both once before and I wasn't eager to repeat the experience.

Years ago, I had an appointment with a girl who trimmed my brows, slapped a stencil over them, and then used a pencil to draw huge, dark eyebrows on my face. I barely recognized myself. I knew I could wash it off when I got home, but my husband, Cameron, didn't know that when I walked through the door. After the shock wore off, he pulled out his phone to show me the TV character I reminded him of; as he searched for a picture online, I envisioned bushy-browed celebs like Brooke Shields, Beyoncé, and Lily Collins.

Then he showed me a picture of Uncle Leo from "Seinfeld."

(Take a moment to Google "Uncle Leo eyebrows Seinfeld" for the visual. I'll wait.)

We still laugh at those brows. And I've heard that the brow studio doesn't use stencils anymore. But you can see why laminating them and having a tint to boot would give me pause.

My girl assured me the results would be fantastic, so I booked an appointment. First, she painted the chemical solution onto my brows, covered them with plastic wrap, and let everything sit for five minutes. Then she brushed a setting solution and tint on to make the brows darker and reminded me the color would begin to fade after a couple of days.

At this point, visions of Uncle Leo danced in my head.

Finally, she trimmed by brows, sat me up, and handed me a mirror. And, gals, I was *in love* with my eyebrows. They were dark, for sure, but they looked so much thicker and healthier. Best of all, it was my hair, just better. They also felt glued in place, nary a straggly hair. She told me to avoid getting them wet and sleeping on my face for a couple of days, but then it would be back to brow business as usual. Because the chemical solution gives the hair shape and hold, I wouldn't have to use gel, but I would have to fill in any gaps with a pencil. Easy peasy.

This time, I wanted to avoid scaring my husband when I got home, so I held my hand over my brows when I saw him and said, "Don't worry. They *will* fade." Then I unveiled The Brows.

"Wow! They're . . . different," he said.

I wasn't fazed, so enamored was I with my pre-'90s look. And just a few hours later, he told me he was used to them. Almost. He admitted the next day that he had to remind himself, "This too shall pass."

But I knew the biggest test would come when I picked my kids up from daycare because they have a knack for spotting anything and everything that happens on my face. In recent weeks, my 3-year-old daughter had noticed when I wore navy eyeliner instead of brown and pointed out a pimple on my cheek. And one night, my 5-year-old son, while holding my face lovingly in his hands, asked me why I had beaver teeth.

Ruthless.

I was expecting them to notice Mom's bushy, dark eyebrows, but neither kid said a thing. Huh. Brow lamination: effective but won't scare your kids.

It's been three weeks since my appointment and the color has faded to a slightly darker-than-normal brown. What I love most is the bushiness, with fluffier hair that stays in place. Getting ready in the morning is quicker, too, because I don't have to use as much pencil for them to look full. Needless to say, I'm sold on lamination.

Brow efforts aside, I've made other changes based on Eldo's recommendations, like not using eye makeup under my eyes and swapping my tinted serum for Armani's Luminous Silk foundation, a magical formulation that keeps my skin looking polished all day. And when my T-zone erupts with oil, I use blotting papers instead of powder. That happens a lot, by the way. The mineral sunblock I apply before my makeup makes my forehead and chin glisten by about noon every day, so I keep those Shiseido papers in my purse 24/7. (Quick check-in here: You're wearing mineral sunblock too, right? If not, be sure to read chapter 2!)

Other techniques, like tapering my eyeliner off at the arch of my eye, aren't going as smoothly. Literally or figuratively. My eyelids are getting more crepe-y and crinkly by the day, so applying eyeliner is tricky. Even if I get a smooth line, I struggle to taper it off mid-eye. It looks so unfinished and awkward that I draw the last bit in every single time.

I gave up on that technique a few months ago and started Googling "eyeliner for crepe-y eyelids." After a bit of poking around—and, whoopsadaisy, a quick detour online to order a pair of sandals for summer—I ended up on Suzanne The Beauty Shaman's YouTube channel. Suzanne Blons is a long-time aesthetician and celebrity makeup artist who's worked with everyone from Hillary Clinton and Jesse Jackson to Christiane Amanpour and Peyton Manning. And as a woman who's a vocal advocate for embracing your age, she's passionate about sharing beauty tips and advice for women over 40.

What caught my attention was her video called "How to do eyeliner for mature women! 5 tips on creating the perfect eyeliner that looks gorgeous!" I immediately hit play.

My friends, those were seven minutes and twenty-one seconds well spent.

Suzanne blew my mind and has completely reversed the order in which I apply my eye makeup. For my entire makeup-wearing life, I'd been applying a lighter shadow on my lid, brushing a darker color into the crease, and drawing eyeliner last. But after watching her video, here are my steps:

1. Apply eyeliner and soften the line with a brush.
2. Brush darker eyeshadow into the crease.
3. Apply lighter eyeshadow on the lid.
4. Blend shadows together.
5. Add mascara.

Applying eyeliner first is genius! You can draw, blend, and even fix it without messing your eyeshadow up. I also loved her tip to hold the pencil from below and apply eyeliner to your top lid from there to stay close to the lashes. I've been using her technique for a few weeks now and find that getting super close to the lash line makes it easier to get a smooth line. Finally, running a thin, slanted brush over the eyeliner helps soften the line and mask any mistakes.

I emailed Suzanne to tell her how much I enjoyed the video and asked if we could speak. That's how we ended up on a virtual chat one afternoon, she from her home base in Boulder, Colorado, and me at my kitchen table. Suzanne told me that after years of working as a professional model and doing makeup in Washington, D.C., for politicians, models, and TV personalities, she was tired of hearing people bash older women and their looks. "I'll be behind the scenes and producers will say about the women I'm working with, 'She looks old. Is there anything else you can do? Can you give her some injections right now?' There are so many criticisms leveled at women."

Suzanne finally had enough. On her YouTube channel, she shares videos to not only show women how to care for their skin and do their makeup but to remind them what an aging woman looks like and empower them to feel good in their skin. And skincare is a big focus. Here's her number-one suggestion: Before applying makeup, make sure you prep the skin with things like vitamin C serums, hyaluronic acid, and moisturizer. Skin that appears plump and full is the perfect foundation for a light- to medium-coverage, um, foundation.

When picking a foundation, she recommends looking for words like "moisturizing" and "nourishing" that indicate a dewy finish, which is a smarter option for older women than full-coverage, matte foundations. "I can't tell you the number of women who say to me, 'I want to cover my wrinkles.' It's like, honey, you don't ever cover them. There's no such animal!"

If you're going to spend more money on a product, concealer is high on her list; she says the cheaper ones settle into fine lines and "look like crap." I should mention here that Suzanne's website has an e-shop with some of her favorite products. She says the biggest mistake women make is slathering concealer everywhere as opposed to applying it where needed. Tapping it into the inner corners of the eyes and just under them is a good strategy, she says. She also suggested I stop applying concealer to my puffy under-eye areas, which only magnifies the issue.

Hot tip: When Suzanne is doing her makeup in the morning, she often spreads a little concealer on her eyelids. "It instantly wakes up my eyes and makes them pop, and then I also fill in my eyebrows because that adds balance to your face." Finally, she adds mascara and lipstick. The routine takes less than five minutes.

But Suzanne says her videos with tips on how to do simple, daytime looks don't get as many views as the ones with more dramatic results; one of her top-viewed tutorials is a Sophia Loren look for aging women. "Older women still want to look amazing!" she says. "I think we have this idea that they just want to look natural and pretty, but there's a side of us that can still be wild and want to get really dressed up without looking garish."

I made a note to check out the Sophia Loren video, along with everything else Suzanne puts out into the world. But what I really wanted to know while we chatted was how she finds her confidence as an aging woman, especially since she's worked for so long in a world that is notorious for scrutinizing and diminishing older women, so I asked her.

"I really go hard on love. It's very hard for women because we're programmed to hate our bodies and to hate aging. I make jokes about aging in my videos because it's good to have a sense of humor about it, but I do work on loving myself. I look in the mirror and say, 'I love you,' as opposed to going, 'My eyes are super puffy today,'" she said. "I try to show up with genuine love for myself and others, because love is what all we want. We want to feel enough. We want to feel accepted. I think those things transcend all the cultural BS that we face as we get older."

Okay. I know I said at the start of the book that I wouldn't tell you to manifest your way to becoming a better you, but Suzanne's answer gave me all the feels. It also motivated me to give that kind of self-love a try. Since chatting with her, I've made a conscious effort to look in the mirror and say, "I love you." On days I need the affirmation most, like when I'm feeling especially tired, puffy, wrinkly, or all the above, I'm sure it helps shift my mindset from frustration to gratitude.

Funny enough, embracing self-acceptance with age is a trait that runs deep among the makeup artists I spoke with. Fatima Thomas is one of them. The Atlanta-raised, New York City–based makeup artist has worked her magic at international fashion shows for brands such as Valentino and DKNY and on celebrities such as Alicia Keys, Jessica Biel, and Whoopi Goldberg. And as a senior, long-time artist with MAC Cosmetics, she's well versed in helping everyday people with their makeup, too.

Now in her early fifties, Fatima told me she wouldn't trade what she's learned and gained as a person just to have the freshness and beauty of her youth. "I'm okay with aging because the alternative means you die. And that's the terminus for everyone, regardless of your skin color, race, socioeconomic status, or position in society. As my grandma used to say, 'We're all going to go to the greedy worms.' For me, it's about quality of life, and the quality of *my* life—especially my inner life—is so much better now. If you can embrace yourself for all your lights and shadows, your triumphs and failures, you come to a place where you can truly love yourself with no conditions."

But there's nothing wrong with wanting to look your best, she adds. We all do. And as someone who applies makeup to people of all ages, ethnicities, and genders, Fatima's beauty philosophy is rooted in the belief that makeup should celebrate and enhance the features people like about themselves. That's an easier job, she says, when someone's been diligent about using—wait for it—sun protection. Fatima does everything she can in the moment to prep skin for makeup application but says it's so much easier when people take care of their skin every day. "When your skin is in good condition, you look vibrant and healthy."

Now, here is my issue. I've been taking care of my skin—especially since interviewing the experts in chapter 2—but there are *so* many days when my skin looks dull in the morning. Whether it's because I'm under-slept or overstressed, "vibrant" is not a word I'd use to describe my face. Fatima had a suggestion.

MAC Cosmetics' bestselling moisturizer, Strobe Cream, has fine, luminescent particles that illuminate the skin. She uses it on clients all the time, but it's also her go-to anytime she feels her skin is dull, like when she's recovering from a cold. She says you can wear it under, over, or mixed with foundation for a subtle glow. And with three shades to choose from—gold, pink, and peach—there's something for everyone.

"Most people I know with brown and deep brown skin prefer the peach or the gold, and I like to use pink on medium and light skin tones," she says. The best way to choose, she says, is to try all three on the back of your hand and see which one you think looks best. No matter what, the cream will all add luminosity and vibrancy. But if in doubt, try the peach. As Fatima explains, "It's a combination of gold and pink, so it's universally flattering on a lot of skin tones."

Something awesome occurred to me just then. As luck would have it—or less luck and more my product-junkie habits—I had a bottle of barely used pink Strobe Cream in my cupboard. I told Fatima that I'd give it a try. The very next morning, I mixed a dollop in with my foundation before applying the mixture to my face.

Babes, glow city.

Now anytime I feel like my skin needs a bit of oomph, I give it the Strobe Cream treatment. I don't know if anyone has noticed the difference, but I think it makes my face look more alive. Thank you, Fatima!

Like any woman who strives to be confident and feel good at any age, Fatima isn't immune to the odd aging-related pet peeve. "If I had any complaint about aging, it's that I want my lips to be as full as they were fifteen years ago," she says. "I can see they're getting a little thinner."

Ah, yes. I'm familiar with this struggle. I told her my lips and the lines around them are my biggest concern, too. I rarely wear lipstick or liner because they seem to accentuate those small lines creeping in above my top lip. Plus, my lips are always dry. For all those reasons, I stick to wearing gloss—but after chatting with Fatima, I'm willing to try something new. See the box below for her favorite lip products and advice on how to use them.

Before we ended our phone call, Fatima said she's happy more and more women are shifting the narrative on what it means to get older. "We have to change how we think about aging. It's

Fatima Thomas's Fave Lip Products

Here are her top picks for anyone wanting to improve their lip looks:

1. MAC **Lip Scrubtious**: "This lip scrub really helps to condition and moisturize your lips."
2. MAC **Prep + Prime Lip**: "It's the No. 1 lip primer in North America. It's like Velcro for your lipstick. Make sure you put it on just outside of your natural lip line and give it 30 seconds to set."
3. MAC **Lip Pencil in Spice**: "Especially if you're getting lines, use lip liner. I prefer a nude like MAC Spice—it's the almighty liner for every woman, person, man, child, you name it. Define your lips with it. And if you like to overdraw them a bit, the lip primer is going to make it easier. Then put on your lip gloss or lipstick. You're good to go."
4. Algenist **GENIUS Liquid Collagen Lip**: "I've used it religiously for a few years. It really penetrates the lips, so I put that on and top it with an emollient-based balm for added moisture."

really about embracing every phase of your life and getting the best out of it."

I am *so* into this mindset. And I must say, it's exciting to hear more and more women say it out loud. I will *not* be spending my midlife years chasing endless ways to look younger—but I do want to look the best I can. And I believe good makeup can help. So can the right attitude, and I'm grateful to women like Fatima and Suzanne for voicing theirs. Because though my whole makeup quest started when I watched the show "Younger," that's not actually my goal. I want to be who I am, be my age, and look good!

On that front, I've realized I feel best when my eyes look refreshed and well defined—no small feat considering I feel groggy and puffy most mornings. Luckily, I've gleaned some helpful tips while chatting with a few other makeup artists, be it while getting my makeup done or interviewing them for background while researching this book. Here are four of their suggestions that have forever changed how I do my eye makeup:

1. **Always tightline your upper waterline.** Our lashes get sparser with age, but tightlining—applying eyeliner to your upper waterline (the watery line of skin between the upper lashes and the eye)—can make them appear thicker and lusher, not to mention make hooded eyes look less droopy. To try this technique, lift your upper eyelid with your non-dominant hand to expose the line of skin underneath your top lashes. Use your dominant hand to run a waterproof pencil or gel eyeliner back and forth, filling the line with color from the outer corner to the inner corner. You can use a soft color, like a dark brown, gray, or taupe, and the line doesn't have to be perfect. You can even push it up into the base of your lashes. Says one artist, "It will make a world of difference even if you're not wearing eyeliner on top."

2. **Apply a brightening eyeliner along your lower waterline to look more awake.** A Calgary-based makeup artist suggested I line my lower waterline with a brightening eyeliner every morning. To do this, sweep an eyeliner back and forth across the line to fill it with a light color; she says white is often too harsh but a nude or off-white suits most people. She swears this technique make her clients' and her own eyes look brighter, more refreshed, and well rested.

3. **Try a "mascara cocktail" to create the ultimate lash look.** Mascaras are typically designed to either volumize and thicken or lengthen your lashes. Why wear just one? A Toronto makeup artist told me she applies both formulas to her clients' lashes for a more dramatic effect. The key is in how you layer them. She applies the volumizing mascara first and as close to the eyelash roots as possible, wiggling her wand up and out. Next, she sweeps the lengthening mascara through the lashes, focusing on mid-lash to the ends. To finish, she sometimes uses a clean wand to define the lashes and remove any clumps.

4. **To amp things up for special occasions or a nighttime look, add half lashes to the outer corners of your eyes.** I'd never heard of half lashes before, but they're just as the name suggests: false lashes that are shorter than a full-length set, so they're more subtle. One artist described them as a little push-up bra for your eyes. Ardell, MAC, and LoveSeen (Jenna Lyons's lash brand) offer half lashes, but you can also just cut any false lashes you already own in half. And if you've ever struggled to apply a full strip of lashes before (um, me too), don't be scared away. The pros say half lashes are easier to handle because there's less length to maneuver and glue.

The half lashes intrigued me.

In my late twenties, I once tried to glue false lashes on my lids for a big night out but gave up after twenty messy, frustrating minutes. Not only could I not get the lashes to stick, but I was surprised I didn't blind myself with glue.

A few years later, and still in want of thick, fluttery eyelashes, I turned to the experts. When a lash clinic opened near my house, I was among the first clients in to get lash extensions. And those lashes were unreal—long, wispy, fun. I felt like a million sexy bucks and loved how quick they made getting ready every morning. But the appointments ultimately ate up too much time and money, so I stopped going.

However, owning a pair of subtle half lashes that I could apply on my own? I was willing to give it a try. First, I jumped on Amazon to peruse my half-lash options. Ardell was out of stock, so I went with a well-reviewed brand called Frihappy. Three pair cost me all of $12. When they showed up at my door the next day, I practically skipped to the bathroom. And then I realized I needed glue. After stopping by a drugstore a few days later to buy a $10 tube of Duo Striplash Adhesive, I was finally ready for my lash experiment.

Let's jump to the pros. Cost-wise, I was thrilled. The half lashes and glue I snagged to give my eyes the promising "push-up bra" effect cost a fraction of what I used to spend. And I could use them many times over.

Now to the cons. The main one being: If you're not skilled with lash application (hi, welcome, happy to have you), half lashes still take some practice to master. But I can attest they *are* easier than full lashes.

On day one, I shocked myself when I was able to stick the lashes to the outer corners of my eyes after just ten minutes of maneuvering with a set of tweezers and my fingers. Here's what helped: looking slightly down into a mirror, using tweezers to place the lashes on my lid and then my fingers to gently push and secure their ends. The results were subpar, though, because I didn't get them close enough to my lash line, leaving a tiny but visible gap between my natural lashes and the false ones.

But, gals, I could see the potential! The half lashes weren't as obvious as a full set but still added drama to my eyes, and they were ultra light on my lids. A little *too* long and fluttery for daily use, they'd be perfect for a night out.

I'd glued the lashes on in the middle of the afternoon—nothing like wearing false lashes while you sit alone at home and fold laundry—so I couldn't wait for my husband to get home from work. He used to love my eyelash extensions, so I was curious to see if he noticed.

He did not.

Granted, there was a lot happening when he walked through the door. I was stirring tomato sauce, and our kids were hurtling through the house at tornado speed, but even when we sat down to eat, no one noticed.

That's how subtle these half lashes were, despite me feeling like they'd be too long for daytime wear. Still, I carefully peeled them off before heading to T-ball practice with my kids and put them back in their container.

Since then, I've found and ordered a popular half-lash set from Ardell and am determined to practice my application technique until I get it right. I'm also excited to experiment with new lash looks when I get all dolled up. That's something I still love to do, although the opportunities to be glam are few and far between. (See: T-ball practice with kids.) I'm now more excited as a 40-something to get ready for a fancy night out than when I was younger *because* it's so rare. On those special occasions, I take my time applying makeup and typically use darker colors I only bust out at night, like navy and deep purple.

But to get some new ideas, I watched Suzanne's tutorial for an updated Sophia Loren look. Essential viewing, in my humble opinion. Not only is her gray-and-black eye makeup stunning, but she shares such helpful tips on how to make it work for mature skin; the advice I took to heart was that I should use a quality eye serum to make sure my whole eye area is hydrated and can handle the dark eyeshadows to come. Why hadn't I—someone who houses the equivalent of a mini-Sephora in her own bathroom—thought of using an eye serum before?

I've always struggled with dryness around my eyes, and the drugstore cream I had been using wasn't super moisturizing. So, within twenty-four hours of watching Suzanne's tutorial—and after doing some research, since the one Suzanne recommends isn't available in Canada—I bought Lancôme Absolue Revitalizing Eye Serum. (This has not been a cheap chapter to pen.) I've been using the serum for a few weeks and notice the skin around my eyes is less puffy and better moisturized, which makes it easier to apply makeup.

And as for Suzanne's Sophia Loren look? I gave it a shot one night before heading out with friends. The trickiest part was—is always!—the eyeliner. I didn't have a gel eyeliner on hand so used my regular black pencil to draw a thin line on my upper lid. Meh. My skills still need work. Thankfully, using a soft, small brush to soften the line with powder helped. But the rest of the look was lovely. A bit dramatic, très chic.

I'd be remiss if I didn't share a few more glamming-up tips I learned from Liz Layton, a Vancouver-based regional education trainer with MAC Cosmetics. And Liz knows glam. She's been backstage at New York Fashion Week and other fashion shows doing makeup for the likes of Giambattista Valli, Dsquared2, Frame, and others; she's prepped models for editorial shoots; and she loves having fun with Halloween makeup. Nuff said.

Liz is in her forties like me—"The struggles are real!" she says with a laugh—and says using a primer after skincare and before makeup is essential at this stage of life. "When you're 22, partying, and you get three hours of sleep, your makeup is still going to look great the next day," she says. "For the rest of us, we may need a little coaxing from our products. Incorporating a good primer can flex what you already use and really influence the way your makeup looks."

Like skincare, primers help plump and hydrate the skin. They can also add radiance, blur imperfections, and help grip makeup for longer wear. There are two MAC versions she recommends: the award-winning Fix + Magic Radiance Primer and Setting Spray, "a mist-on moisturizer that preps and hydrates," and the newer Studio Radiance Moisturizing + Illuminating Silky Primer, "a watery gel primer that hydrates and makes the skin look and feel so juicy."

In addition to applying a primer before foundation, Liz loves to amp luminosity for a night out. She taps highlighter cream onto three spots: the apples of the cheeks, the center of the eyelids, and the middle of the eyebrow bones just underneath the brows. "Think of it as a line you want to create," she says. "So when your face turns in the light, you get a hit of light around your eye area."

And don't forget about your body! If your outfit is showing skin, Liz suggests adding a bit of shine, be it on your collarbone,

Liz Layton's Essential Brushes

As a long-time makeup artist with MAC Cosmetics, Liz has roughly fifty brushes at her beauty station. But we don't need that many. Here are the three essentials she always recommends:

1. **A foundation brush:** "It should have a good bristle density so you can buff and polish. I love a good foundation brush because you can also use it for your powder, blush, and anything that needs to be tapped and blended."
2. **An eyeliner brush:** "Get one you can use with your powder shadows to transform them into eyeliners because that's a simple way to add a little bit of drama to your look."
3. **A rounded eyeshadow brush:** "You want something fluffy that you're able to blend with. Whether it's casting a light layer all over your lid or working color through the crease, a rounded brush that fits your eye shape is a really good tool. You can also use it for concealer and highlighting, as well."

shoulders, fronts of the legs, or wherever. "If you spend all your time making sure the skin on your face looks its best, but you're dry and ashy from the neck down, it's not as cute, right?" To get that luminosity onto the body, Liz says any moisturizer with a pearly finish will do. Or you can do as she does: get a travel-sized pot of moisturizer from the drugstore and stir some loose, shimmery powder into it. Even if it's a pigment you wear on your eyes, the mixture will be perfect for your body, too.

Last, Liz told me her eyeliner rule: Stay away from wearing black eyeliner during the day so you can reserve its use for a special occasion. "In general, it's hard to go any darker than black for drama!" she says, which is why it's so effective for a night out.

Shortly after speaking with the experts about how to get glammed up, I received an invitation to a black-tie gala in Calgary. I hadn't been to a fancy event in ages, so I decided to get my makeup done at the Nordstrom beauty counter near me. And it was wild watching my lovely makeup artist, Nowreen Ali, put nearly every tip I'd recently learned into action.

First, she prepped my skin with a luxe Sisley Black Rose Cream Mask and Sisley Eye Contour Mask. Then she pressed La Mer's ultra-rich Crème de la Mer Moisturizing Cream onto my face. The makeup wizardry that ensued was a blur, but a few steps stood out, like when Nowreen buffed Dior Airflash Spray Foundation onto my face with a dense Dior foundation brush; used balm on my lips before *and* after applying Charlotte Tilbury's famous Pillow Talk lipstick; swirled the two lightest colors from Charlotte's Pillow Talk Dreams eyeshadow palette onto my lids; and lined my upper lid with a deep brown pencil. Last, she misted a setting spray onto my face and had me rub Tom Ford Soleil Blanc Shimmering Body Oil onto my décolletage.

After looking at myself in the mirror, I had one question for Nowreen: Could she pretty please come to my house every morning and do my makeup?

The results were *that* impressive. My skin was dewy and plump, the green in my hazel eyes popped more than usual, and even my lips looked fuller. Magic, I tell you. Did anyone else notice the magic that night? I have no idea. But it didn't matter, really, because I felt incredibly confident at the gala, like a superhero in a glittery dress and heels. Nowreen's skillful application made me feel like the best version of myself. And *that* is makeup's true superpower.

Unfortunately, hiring a makeup artist on the daily isn't in my budget, so I must fend for myself. But with all the tips and tricks I've learned from the pros, I'm slowly improving my game. Every morning I make sure to fill my brows, tightline my upper waterlines with a dark brown pencil, fill my lower waterlines with a nude-colored liner, and prep my skin with an illuminating primer (wet n wild's Photo Focus Dewy Face Primer is my new fave—and it's so affordable!). For night, I use the Charlotte Tilbury palette I could not leave Nordstrom without, apply black or dark gray eyeliner, and add a radiant moisturizer to my shoulders, chest, and legs.

The results aren't even close to Nowreen's, but I'm digging these tweaks for making me feel more vibrant. As we all know, that feeling is what matters most. As Eldo told me, "I want to think that if someone is taking the time to wear makeup, they're doing it for themselves and not for someone else."

And that, ladies, is the whole, massive point. We are aging, but we don't need to conform to anyone's idea of how we should look or act. We don't need to blend in, wear only neutral-toned makeup, or disappear into the sunset because we're over 40. We are not invisible. We are bold, beautiful, rebellious beings who can master Sophia Loren makeup and slick their shoulders with glowy moisturizer and flip their middle fingers at the idea that older women aren't sexy or cool.

Who's with me?

And who's ready to experiment with all these makeup tips? We all deserve to feel fantastic as we get ready in the morning or for a special night out. With that in mind, here's a cheat sheet with a few reminders on how to put your best face forward.

THE CHEAT SHEET

- Use nourishing skincare, sun protection, and, depending on the look you're going for, a primer to prep the skin for makeup. And don't forget to protect and moisturize your lips, too.
- If you don't own them yet, invest in a good foundation brush, an eyeliner brush, and a round, fluffy eyeshadow brush.
- Use a light- to medium-coverage foundation with descriptors like "moisturizing" and "radiant" for a dewier finish and add concealer sparingly. When oil strikes, use blotting papers.
- Avoid wearing eye makeup on or below your lower lashes, which will help keep the focus up—a good thing for us aging gals.
- Even if you apply no other makeup, fill in your brows. They give the face structure and, again, help keep the focus up.
- For an easy daytime look, try adding a bit of concealer to your eyelids to make your eyes pop and don't forget to tightline your upper waterline to make lashes appear thicker. Fill your lower waterline with a brightening liner if you're feeling tired. Add mascara and you're set.
- For nighttime looks, add more luminosity to your face and body with creams or highlighters, glue half lashes to the outer corner of your eyes, and apply black eyeliner. Now go have fun!
- Look in the mirror and say "I love you" every day. Come on, do it! Self-love breeds happiness and true beauty.

CHAPTER FOUR

Rethink the Friendships You Have and the Ones You Want to Have

In my late thirties, I noticed something that made me feel sad and unsure about my place in the world: I was drifting away from some of my oldest friends. The shift in our friendships was slow and subtle but a shock to my system, all the same.

Many of us had been intertwined in each other's lives for decades. We grew up, studied, traveled, and partied together. We bounded through our twenties together, moving cities, changing jobs, and pursuing new ambitions. My world had revolved around my friends, a mix of girls and guys I hung out with all the time. To then feel myself drifting apart from a group that felt like family was painful. It's still hard. Some days, I miss how things used to be, how easy our friendships were to nourish and sustain when we were young. How central we were in each other's lives.

But the evolution was probably inevitable.

Our friendships have changed in adulthood because our lives have changed. And I would never bemoan the tremors that shifted the foundation of our relationships because they came on the heels of life events that were natural, exciting, and filled with hope. Some of us got married, some stayed single. Some had kids, others adopted dogs. There were promotions, divorces, travels, new homes in far-away neighborhoods. You know, all the usual stuff that happens on the road to midlife.

And while we were growing as individuals and venturing down our different paths, each of us established friendships outside the group. I know I did—and I am so grateful to have the friends I made during those years. Some of my closest pals today are the ones I met in my late twenties and thirties while I was working, exercising at my gym, and, in one case, volunteering to make dinner for homeless families. I feel lucky to have forged such solid friendships in adulthood.

Still, navigating my older friendships has been one of the hardest things about midlife. It's been especially difficult since one girls' night out a few years ago when tension exploded between friends, creating a divide that hasn't yet healed. In the aftermath, our group has rearranged itself into different alignments and social circles. I was not in the center of that storm, so I see friends from both sides every now and then, albeit some more than others.

But things are certainly different than before. And as I see some of my old friends less and less, I wonder: Will my forever friends be in my life forever? Should I do everything I can to keep my old friendships alive, or am I better off prioritizing the few people I connect with? And the big one: Am I a good friend?

Those are the questions on my mind lately. And as I consider their answers, I spend a lot of time thinking about how to invest my time and energy into my long-standing relationships. Honestly, I spend a lot of time thinking about how to invest my time and energy into *all* my friendships. I love my friends dearly and want to be the best friend I can, now and always.

But maintaining adult friendships is tricky—if for no other reason than we are all so overscheduled and tired at the end of the day. Every year my responsibilities loom bigger than before while my free time dwindles. My friends have equally demanding lives with their jobs, partners, families, and interests. Still, we do our best to prioritize time with each other.

At the end of every get-together, we pull out our phones to compare calendars, scheduling dinners weeks ahead of time, knowing there's still a good chance someone will have to cancel because of work, a sick kid, or general life overload. We plan the odd weekend away. We text each other memes, life updates, and texts that say, "Miss you! Can't wait to see you soon."

Alas, friendship in my forties sometimes feels like I'm in long-distance relationships with people in my city.

On top of all that, I occasionally meet a woman I click with and would love to hang out with more. Such a magical feeling in adulthood, no? There's an inherent barrier stopping us from nurturing a new friendship, though. Time. There just isn't enough of it.

I take solace knowing I'm not alone as I wrestle with prioritizing my friendship efforts. Far from it. Women in my circle talk about how their long-standing friend groups have struggled to stay together, especially now that they're in their forties. Sometimes there are clear reasons, other times not. One friend mentioned her group of friends from college recently split in two over a blow-up about differing parenting views. Another said she's not sure she'd be friends with some old pals if they met today because they've become such different people in adulthood. And another told me she's drifted from a few of her close friends but doesn't know why.

It's safe to say many of us are navigating something within our friendships in midlife. To help us through, I called upon two renowned friendship experts, Dr. Marisa G. Franco and Shasta Nelson, to learn how and why friendships often change for women at this stage of life—and what we can do to nurture the best friendships possible.

Before we get into their brilliant insights and advice, let me tell you about these experts and why I was excited to speak with them.

Marisa is the *New York Times* bestselling author of *Platonic: How the Science of Attachment Can Help You Make—and Keep—Friends*. She's also a psychologist, speaker, professor at the University of Maryland, and contributor to *Psychology Today*, among other publications. I'd been following her on Instagram (@drmarisagfranco) for her quick and genius tips—including how to deepen friendships, have better conversations with our friends, and shift our perspective on conflict—so I was thrilled when she agreed to a phone conversation.

Shasta is a California-based speaker, go-to media resource, and the author of three books, including *Frientimacy: How to Deepen Friendships for Lifelong Health and Happiness*. She has also interviewed or polled nearly 10,000 women about friendship; as an interviewer, I can confirm that represents a *massive amount* of acquired knowledge. Shasta is passionate about helping people establish and maintain meaningful friendships in adulthood. I couldn't wait to glean her wisdom during our phone call and learn how we gals can boost our frientimacy skills.

Given their research, expertise, and personal experiences, I asked both experts to set the scene for us. What often happens with women's friendships during midlife?

"Definitely friends going through different life stages or ebbing and flowing in their level of connection," Marisa says.

Ah, yes, I can relate. The ebb and flow are palpable.

I told her about how the dynamics in my oldest friend group have shifted and my uncertainty about my place in the new landscape. Her advice to me and everyone: Don't write off friendships just because they're in the ebb.

She points to a study that found when people in a long-distance friendship see their connection as flexible but not fragile, their friendship sustains more. She says having that mentality can benefit all friendships, long-distance or not. "If your friendship is in the ebb, don't assume it's over. Assume that it's going through its natural cycle, and there will be a time in which you can reconnect. If you assume, 'Our friendship is no more,' you won't reach out, and it will become a self-fulfilling prophecy."

Noted. And more on what I did with her advice later.

Aside from friends experiencing varying levels of connection, Marisa says another phenomenon happens as we age thanks to the socio-emotional selectivity hypothesis.

Ah, yes, I can relate. The socio-emotional selectivity hypothesis is palpable.

Joking. I had no idea what that meant when I heard it, either.

In essence it means we become pickier about our friends as we age. As Marisa explains, socio-emotional selectivity hypothesis is "a term that basically means we select our friends based off the needs that we have in life at a given time. Younger people are looking to expand their identities, so they have more friends. People in middle age and beyond are starting to think about the time they have left and want to spend it with people that are meaningful connections to them."

If you haven't made meaningful connections yet and worry you won't ever find those close friendships, don't worry, Marisa says. There are plenty of ways to make new friends in adulthood—and we would *all* do well to give them a go. Because no matter our friend history or status, friendships are forever evolving.

Shasta told me even people who belonged to a strong friend group when they were younger can experience upheaval in midlife.

"One of the big things that happens in midlife is that we *had* good friends, so we keep thinking we need them. But we aren't really relying on them anymore. We're not calling them. We're not talking to them very often," Shasta says. "And a loneliness often creeps up in our thirties, especially because most of us feel like we had good friends in school, but then we got really busy and started doing life."

All of that accelerates as we head into our forties, a stage when doing life typically results in women prioritizing work, family, and other caregiver responsibilities but letting our friendships slide, often without us realizing it's happening. Slowly, we can lose touch, drift apart, and feel disconnected.

It's a common issue for everyone these days and one that can't be pinned on having a specific personality type. As Shasta wrote in *Frientimacy*, "Even the most extraverted and outgoing among us know the pain of wishing we had closer friends. Research suggests that most of us replace half our closest friends every seven years; at that rate, basically anyone experiencing life change will experience some friendship losses and transitions, many times over."

The seven-year stat stunned me. But it also made me feel . . . relieved. Friendship transitions are normal, expected even.

That said, the turnover rate is surprising.

I asked Shasta if the stat shocks other people. Yes, she says audiences are skeptical when she talks about it onstage. But to help put it into perspective, she asks everyone in the room to consider which five people they'd ask to be in their bridal party today. She then asks, who would they have asked seven years ago? Chances are two or three of them are not the same people. "As soon as I say *that,* everyone's like, 'Oh, yeah . . .'"

One of the most powerful reminders in that stat, she says, is that certain relationships in our lives will lose their urgency and significance—for reasons as small as we don't work together anymore, or our kids no longer attend the same school—so we should all be in the game of building new friendships. "If you believe in the research, you always want to be building the friend pipeline," she says, "and be mindful of the fact you need to be making new friends at different levels that can continue to grow in their importance."

And make no mistake, friendships should be paramount. Not a nice-to-have in our lives, a must-have. Here are just a few of the reasons we should all prioritize our friendships during midlife and beyond:

1. **Friendships improve our happiness, health, and longevity.** Being married and being a mother are incredibly meaningful roles many women have in midlife. But those relationships are often the most stressful ones in our lives, says Shasta, at least because of how we "do life" right now. Friends, on the other hand, not only boost our happiness, but they also act as a protective barrier to our health. Marisa agrees. She says, "Your social network affects your longevity even more than your diet and how much you exercise. And the impact of social connection on your health actually tends to increase over time. So, if you're older, friends only become more important."
2. **Having friends benefits our romantic relationships, too.** The mental health of you and your spouse are intertwined, so anything you do to improve yours will improve your spouse's. Marisa says one study found that once you make a friend, not only are you less depressed, but your spouse also becomes less depressed. In addition, studies have found that friends help us regulate our emotions, become more resilient to stress within our marriages, and release less stress hormone when we face relationship difficulties. "Sometimes we think of friends and spouses as antagonistic, like, 'You're spending time with your friends and not spending time with me,'" she says. "It's more like, 'You're spending time with your friends, and that means we're going to have more quality time when we spend time together.'"
3. **Prioritizing friendships gives us the opportunity to model ideal behavior for our kids.** Many mothers feel like they must spend every moment with their kids, says Shasta, and only see friends when it won't interfere with them. They'll grab a drink with friends after their kids go to bed, for example, or only meet friends when kids are in school. But doing that means we never show our kids

> that stepping out of our lives to be with our friends is valuable. Simple things like telling our kids we're going to meet a friend for coffee, going away for a girls' weekend, or hosting dinner for friends in our homes allow us to model what good friendship behavior looks like. And seeing our efforts will help our kids develop necessary friendship skills of their own. Shasta says, "We need to realize that having friendships makes you a good mom."

And I'll add my reason to the list: Friends make life more fun in ways big and small. My close friends make me laugh, plan adventures for us, support me through my lows, celebrate my highs, send me recipes and articles they know I'll love, give the best hugs, and make my world brighter with their mere presence.

To sum up, not only are friends like harbingers of happiness, they benefit our health, increase our longevity, and improve our relationships with other loved ones.

So. Now that we've established why friends *should* play a leading role in our lives, what can we do in midlife to make the most of our friendships?

A wise first step, say the experts, is to stop and assess our current friend situation. We cruise through life at warp speed, so pausing to consciously audit how our friendships are going (or not) in adulthood and tapping into how we feel about them will help us focus our friendship efforts.

Sounds easy enough, but it's not so simple. Unlike how we can monitor things like muscle gain to gauge whether our fitness plan is working, we don't have a concrete measurement system or tool to evaluate our friendships. Not to worry—the experts have us covered with questions to guide our reflection. Answering them honestly and with self-awareness, says Marisa, is "how you can be very discerning and steer your connections in ways wherein you're going to keep friendships that are really restorative and fulfilling to you."

Let's get to them. In the coming days, set aside some time to reflect on the following nine questions I've compiled from Shasta and Marisa:

- What do my friendships look like today?
- What have they been like in the past?
- Who are the people that are actually supporting me right now?
- How loved do I feel?
- Who's doing life with me?
- When I look back, who are the people I really connected to?
- Who are the people I didn't?
- What qualities in my friends do I want to keep in my life?
- Am I hungry for more connection?

To prepare for this exercise, prompt insightful answers, and dig deeper into the quality of your friendships, it might help to keep Shasta's "frientimacy" requirements in mind. Intimacy in friendships, she says, is established when three essential things exist in the relationship: positivity, consistency, and vulnerability. Here's how she writes about the impact of each in *Frientimacy:*

- *For us to feel satisfied, we must feel our interaction is rewarding, practicing positivity with each other.*
- *For us to feel safe, we must feel some level of trust, practicing consistency with each other.*
- *For us to feel seen, we must be willing to reveal ourselves, practicing being vulnerable with each other.*

This resonates with me, as the strongest friendships in my life have all three elements in spades. We are consistent and see, text, or talk to each other often, or at least enough to know what's happening in each other's lives. We're open with each other, revealing our insecurities and struggles, and don't just give the glossy, high-level updates of our best moments. And we are always positive with each other; I leave our hangouts feeling higher on life than before.

In fact, I'd say positivity is my number-one requirement in a friend. Over the last twenty years, I've slowly filtered out people who were too negative, judgmental, and critical when we were together. I've also done the same with people who show no reciprocal interest in my life—a trait I've found beyond deflating in some old friendships and a few of my previous romantic partners. I gravitate to people who ask questions and show genuine interest in what's happening with me, and I aim to deliver the same in return.

But Shasta's extensive polling reveals many women are not getting enough positivity from their friendships, as they consistently give that element the lowest score out of the three. Sadly, their scoring does not bode well for their relationships. Positivity is the basic requirement for friendship, says Shasta, because if we're not enjoying each other, we won't want to be consistent with each other or feel loved enough to be vulnerable. And our friendships will suffer, even crumble. It's as simple as that. "As women," she says, "positivity is definitely the area we need to work on the most."

As evidence, she points to a finding from American psychologist John Gottman that says the positivity in our relationships must outweigh the negativity by a ratio of 5:1. That means anytime we experience disappointment, conflict, stress, or heartache in a friendship, we need at least five positive experiences to recover. Shasta writes in *Frientimacy*, "Relationships that drop below that 5:1 ratio will erode and eventually collapse, while relationships with a high joy:pain ratio will flourish."

Fortunately, boosting the positivity in our relationships isn't hard. Nor does the effort demand a bunch of energy. Shasta says it can be as easy as commenting on a friend's social media post, remembering her birthday, texting the day after a hangout to say how much fun you had, voicing how proud you are of her accomplishments, or asking her about her life. Doing the above will raise the positivity bar, leave your friend feeling good, and help your friendship flourish.

"Our number-one job as a friend should be making sure this person leaves my presence feeling better about themselves, and feeling confident that I love them, support them, and have a good time with them," she says. Though we may think our love for our friends is obvious, we can never go wrong by reaffirming it. "One of the greatest gifts we can give to our friends is the reminder that they are our friends, and we like them."

Using the positivity, consistency, and vulnerability lens to consider your answers to the experts' nine questions is bound to unearth some realizations. As in, you may be totally content with your friendships. You might be lonely and hungry for stronger, deeper connections. You may want to make new friends or reconnect with ones you've drifted from. You might choose to do both, investing in your highest-quality friendships while seeking new ones. And it may even be time to let go of the friendships that no longer serve you.

Ending a friendship is a huge decision, so I asked the experts how we know when it's time to walk away. As Marisa mentioned, friendships ebb and flow, so if yours is in an ebb, she suggests taking a step back and looking at the bigger picture, the pros and cons of your friendship. "Ask yourself, 'Is this a chapter of our book or has it always been the book? Have we always had this issue, and I've pushed it aside—like they've never really asked me questions or been interested in my life—or is this more of a recent development?' Sometimes an ebb can be explained by a certain event, life transition, or differences in friends' lives." If we have evidence that our friend has loved us and been there for us in the past, says Marisa, it's most likely worth sticking it out to see if the friendship can switch from an ebb to a flow.

Shasta echoed the sentiment. Her rule of thumb is the more you've invested in a relationship, confided in that person, and felt close to that friend, the more you owe it to yourself and the other person to try to repair and protect the friendship. Because if we were to walk away anytime we experienced something uncomfortable, awkward, or painful with our friends—or just because we weren't at a high point—we'd start over all the time and never develop deep relationships. She adds, "And we do score happier when we have some people from our past in our lives."

That doesn't mean we have to keep *every* historical friendship, though. It just means salvaging a relationship that has been meaningful and brought us joy in the past is often well worth the effort. To do that, Shasta suggests talking with your friend to address whatever you're feeling or needing, be it more consistency, less judgment, better support. Spending an awkward hour or two with that person to build on the investment you've made over the years will be more fulfilling more quickly, she says, than starting from scratch with someone new. But if you still do not get what you need, it's time for an honest assessment. Shasta says, "If you don't feel supported, safe, and loved in your friendship, it may be time to accept reality and lower your expectations."

Shasta's word choice, innocuous as it may seem, hit me hard. I expected her to say it may be time to accept reality and end the friendship. Say goodbye. Kick that friend to the curb. But it never occurred to me that I could *lower my expectations* of a friendship and keep that person in my life, albeit in a lesser way than before.

This strikes me as an elegant solution for maintaining friendships with people I've grown apart from, for example, but always will adore because we have a shared history. In those situations, I don't feel compelled to discuss or reinvigorate the kind of friendship we had in our twenties. Instead, I'm into the idea of seeing each other when we can—even if it's once a year over coffee, on a girls' weekend, or at a Christmas party—and enjoying those moments for what they are. No labels on our friendship, no expectations, just appreciation for the time we share.

Not all friendships deserve saving, though, especially ones we feel are toxic, unhealthy, and unsafe. When friendships veer into that territory, says Marisa, often there's an uneven dynamic at play. Telltale signs: when one person fulfills their needs at the expense of the other person's or tries to bring the other person down. Sometimes it's obvious the dynamic is unhealthy, like if you fight often or your friend is malicious toward you, but other times it's more subtle. If a friend consistently makes you feel judged, doesn't care about how you feel, brings your energy down, or neglects you, those are valid issues—and they're worth addressing with your friend.

But if nothing changes after your conversation and you decide it's time to end the friendship, Marisa says the kindest thing you can do is tell the person directly, especially if you've been friends for a while. As she told the hosts of the Dear Shandy podcast, "If you don't give someone closure, you trigger something in them called ambiguous loss, which is when someone's grief process is disrupted because they don't have any reason or closure as to why the relationship ended."

Being brave enough to break up with a friend and give them the closure they need to move on sounds doable in theory but terrifying in reality. How do you tell someone you don't want to be friends anymore? As she shared on the podcast, here's the essence of how Marisa would tell a friend it's over: "Lately I've been feeling like we're not as compatible as friends anymore. I've been feeling like we've developed different values and are evolving in different directions. And I just want to make sure you have my transparency that I don't think that this friendship will continue to work for me."

Tough for you to say in the moment, she says, but the best way to help someone understand, grieve the loss of your relationship, and move on.

Hearing Marisa's advice brought back a flurry of feelings from the one time I ended a friendship—a hard but necessary decision in my early thirties. My friend had been in my life since junior high, but she hadn't been showing much interest in my life. Our in-person interactions were often one-sided and left me unfulfilled. On a walk one day, I summoned my courage and told her how I'd been feeling and why, and how much I hoped we could get back to a better place. Sadly, nothing changed over the following months and our friendship fell away.

Looking back on that experience, I feel good knowing I spoke to her about what I needed from our friendship and gave our relationship time to see how things would go. But where I failed, I'm almost certain, is not having a final conversation. My memory is terrible, but I'm 95 percent sure I didn't tell her the friendship wasn't going to work for me, in the end. From what I can remember and the few email exchanges I still have from that time, it seems like we both let the friendship fade in its final months—perhaps a sign she felt it was time to move on, too. I hope that's the case and that she is happy, fulfilled, and thriving these days. I think about her, now and then, and always wish her well.

And though I'm loosening my grip on a few other relationships from my past, I want to reinvest in others. Because after reflecting on my answers to the experts' guiding questions, I want to reinvigorate a few of my most meaningful historical friendships—even if they need some TLC. And I own up to the fact that some of the drifting we've experienced is on me. When I began to feel like I wasn't in the mix as much as I used to be with my old friends, I reached out less, creating the self-fulfilling prophecy Marisa mentioned.

Ultimately, I want to focus on doing two things: nourishing my most loving and supportive relationships, including those from my past that are worth the effort, and establishing and nurturing new friendships with a few women I've recently met. Having the tools to accomplish both is important not just for me but for you, too, because no matter our unique friendship situations, these skills will help us build better friendship futures for ourselves.

Let's start building the toolbox with tips on how to make new friends in midlife and bust a myth while we're at it. Contrary to popular belief, midlife is actually a great time to expand your social circle. Why? Because we're more mature. We know ourselves better. We've seen a few things and been through some shit. Most of us better understand what has and hasn't worked in our past relationships, friendships and otherwise. And we have accrued a wealth of self-knowledge, which helps us assess our wants and needs from our friendships and sustains our relationships in ways we may not expect.

"Developing a sense of self is important for friendship because it's like you have skin instead of a raw nerve. When someone rejects you, and you have a greater sense of self, it won't hit you so deeply at your core," Marisa says. Being older and wiser should then, in theory, help us weather the pain points that inevitably pop up in relationships. "Having time to develop that sense of self means you might have more resilience to some of the dings that come with connection."

Midlife is also a time of transition for many people, she says, and change often creates a sense of loneliness. That means anyone starting a new job, going through a divorce, moving to a different city, retiring from work, or weathering any significant life change will be more open to a new friendship. Focusing on befriending and connecting with "transition-ers" is a smart move, says Marisa, if you'd like to make new friends.

Here are a few more of the experts' top tips on how to expand your social circle and make friends in midlife:

1. **If you pursue a hobby, activity, or interest alone, explore ways to pursue it with others.** You may need to research

options online or ask friends for recommendations, but finding a group that meets regularly, be it for pottery classes, professional development events, or running nights, is key for making new friends. You'll meet new people with similar interests, and the regular meetings will help cement the foundation of your new friendship. As Marisa says, "You're a lot more likely to be successful if you set up something repeated over time versus a one-off." Seeing each other consistently establishes trust, increases knowledge, and builds familiarity. And thanks to the exposure effect, which is our unconscious tendency to like people familiar to us and for them to like us, says Marisa, people we see repeatedly are more likely to respond well to a potential new friendship.

2. **When you join a new community or group, introduce yourself to people.** Seems obvious enough, but it's easy to show up physically and check out mentally. If you're on your phone, only talking to the one person you know, or standing off in the corner, you won't make new connections. "Don't avoid people just because you're nervous or scared," Marisa says. And when you feel that way, remember that people like you more than you think. For real. According to research on the liking gap, says Marisa, people consistently underestimate how liked they are when interacting with others. She also says other research has found that when people are told they will go into a group and be accepted, they become warmer, friendlier, more open. And it becomes a self-fulfilling prophecy, even though they weren't any more likely to be accepted than anyone else. Marisa says, "Assume people like you going into social interactions."

3. **Understand it takes time and effort to establish a friendship.** Shasta points to a University of Kansas study that

> found it takes about fifty hours of time together to move from acquaintance to casual friend, ninety hours to progress from casual friend to friend, and more than two hundred hours to become a close friend. Whatever the exact numbers, Shasta says, "the point is it takes massive hours to build familiarity, even if you click with someone and could be best friends." That's why making the effort to plan consistent hangouts and meet up regularly with new friends stacks the odds in your favor. And it *is* an effort. "Friendships doesn't happen organically in adulthood," Marisa says. "People who think it does are lonelier over time, and people who think it takes effort are less lonely. So, if you don't have the connections you want and you're being passive, your life is likely not going to change on its own. Formulate a plan, join something repeated over time, and reach out to people."

There's no way around it—everything comes back to time, the inherent barrier I mentioned. We all know it's hard to find massive hours for friendships when our lives are already brimming with commitments. That's why I loved Marisa's excellent suggestion on how to find time to see friends: Ask them to join you for things you're doing throughout your day anyway. Going to a group workout? Invite her along. Heading to the farmers' market? Great opportunity to catch up while you shop. Working at a café? Turn your friend into your colleague. "There are so many ways we can be more creative about how we spend our day without adding extra time to what we're doing already and still be able to spend more time deepening our relationships," she says.

Now that we've put a few tools in our toolbox with tips on how to make new friends and find time to invest in those relationships, let's round it out with advice on how to be a great friend. Because, as I told both Shasta and Marisa, evaluating the quality of my friendships is one thing; knowing how to show up as the best friend I can is another. How does it all start with us, and what we can do to make our friends feel safe, supported, and loved?

Ask them, suggests Marisa. She herself has taken that advice from Dr. Kory Floyd, a professor at Arizona State University known for his research on the communication of affection in close relationships, who suggests asking your friends, "What is your favorite way for me to show you how much I appreciate you?" It's like asking their love language but friendship-style. Need a refresher on the five love languages? They are words of affirmation, acts of service, receiving gifts, quality time, and physical touch. Physical touch might be an odd one for friends—although, as I mentioned, I love my friends' hugs. Marisa says she's always surprised when she hears her friends' answers. "I'm like, 'Oh, you're acts of service! Here I am telling you you're amazing when I should be picking you up at the airport.'"

Shasta has another tip. Aside from being positive and communicating to our friends how much we love and support them, which should be baseline behaviors as a friend, she suggests focusing on your role in upholding consistency. One of the most common complaints she hears from women is that they're always the ones inviting friends out, planning get-togethers, initiating communication. If you're not prone to initiating or inviting, she says, then give it a try occasionally or at least thank your friends for playing that role. "Tell your friends, 'I love that you always call me. I want to be better at doing that. You are the one holding us together, so thank you for doing that,'" says Shasta. "Express appreciation for your friends and give them the credit they deserve."

Another hot tip: Pay attention to the "diagnostic moments" in your relationships. Marisa defines these moments as ones that people use to diagnose the health of their friendships—and they tend to occur in very high or very low life moments. These moments should be your cue to step up as a friend. On the high side, when your friend gets a promotion or wins an award, make sure to voice your pride, congratulate them, and take time to celebrate their success. And when a friend is sick or loses a loved one, drop off food or a Starbucks card and check in often to see how they're doing. Our brains remember things more when they're emotionally laden, says Marisa, so they tend to disproportionately affect our memories of moments in the friendship. Bottom line: Don't be passive when diagnostic moments happen. As Marisa says, "Those moments should set off an alarm bell telling you to kick into active friend mode."

Last, give your friends the real, behind-the-scenes view of your life. Both Shasta and Marisa mentioned how critical it is for us to be vulnerable and open with our friends. We can start by nixing the answer, "I'm fine," when our friends ask how we are (unless you really, truly are just fine). Tell them what's going on, whether you're stressed, worried about work, going through something with your partner. Don't always joke about or hide what's really going on in your life. "Being vulnerable and sharing our low moments with our friends can create a lot of intimacy," says Marisa, adding that when we take the lead to be more vulnerable, our friends feel more comfortable to be the same.

To foster even more intimacy, Marisa encourages us to ask our friends questions outside of our usual conversational scripts. She says sometimes friends will go years without talking about a certain thing or delving into an important topic just because no one has asked the question. If you need help busting out of your usual conversational ruts and finding novel questions, consider buying any of the following Marisa-approved items: The Friendship Edition of Koreen Odiney's game, We're Not Really Strangers, designed to deepen existing connections with the friends you consider besties; Esther Perel's game Where Should We Begin—A Game of Stories, which includes prompting questions and story cards to inspire you to share the stories you rarely tell; or Kat Vellos's Better Conversations Calendar, which Marisa brought into her workplace to inspire more intimate conversations with colleagues.

After speaking with Marisa, I immediately hunted down The Friendship Edition of We're Not Really Strangers online and ordered it. (You don't need to ask me twice to shop online.) Most importantly, I didn't waste any time giving my interviewees' tips a try.

Here's a glimpse of what went down with my pals over the coming weeks and months, divided by friend category for your reading pleasure:

Up-and-Coming Friends

To help foster budding friendships, I grabbed our toolbox and unpacked some tools to encourage my nascent relationships to grow and thrive.

First, I've been making a point to invite a fellow mom I clicked with at her son's birthday party to join me for classes at a gym we both love—an easy way to squeeze in a visit without adding something new to our days. Now, whenever I sign up, I send a text to see if she can make it, and she does the same. Our time to connect before and after each class is minimal, but we are seeing each other quasi-consistently, establishing greater familiarity, and enjoying each other's company. (Well, I can't speak for her, but I've been enjoying our chats!) In recent weeks, we've had a couple of play dates with our kids and we're planning a girls' night out soon. Encouraging steps, indeed.

Second, as I considered which qualities I want in my life—and the people in my life that have them—something became obvious: A few acquaintances I highly enjoy, respect, and admire are already orbiting in my world. I just haven't seen them often enough. So, I've taken the reins, inviting them to brunch, organizing outings, planning dinner. Knowing friendships don't happen organically in adulthood, I'm down to make the effort and see if our relationships can blossom into something more.

I should add a caveat here. I am a naturally outgoing and friendly person, so extending myself has not been hard. But I know being vulnerable and reaching out is not an easy task for many people. If you're someone who's nervous to instigate, I hope the experts' tips encourage you to get out there, introduce yourself, and make connections. New friendships await!

As for my few newish relationships, time—and effort, we can't forget about the effort!—will tell. But I'm hopeful at least one or two of these potential friendships will stick. Not because my current friendships are lacking, but because I've come to understand nothing is static. I am changing. We, as women, are changing. Our friendships are changing. And with change comes opportunities for growth, connection, new experiences. I'm investing in friendships at every level to ensure my friend future is bright.

Dear Friends Now

I'm proposing we start using a grown-up version of Best Friends Forever, or BFFs: Dear Friends Now, or DFNs. Given everything we've learned from the experts, it's hard to know what paths our relationships will take. But I *am* sure of one thing: The closest friends I have in my life right now, my most meaningful, loving, and supportive DFNs, are ones I will fight to the death to keep.

I've told my friends I love and appreciate them before, but ever since interviewing Shasta and Marisa, I've ramped up my proclamations. I express my feelings in person. Over text. Via email. No hangout is too insignificant or quick for me to take the opportunity to thank my friends for being my friends. For instance, after a quick happy-hour drink with my dear friends Haithem and Eric the other day, I sent a text: "I love you guys and am so blessed you're in my world." After a night out with Samantha, I wrote: "Love you and am grateful for you." And to Christina, a simple: "Love you, my friend."

Love is my lead, these days. But I'm just trying to do my number-one job and leave my friends feeling more loved than before we spent time together.

As for diagnostic moments? There haven't been many since I've spoken with Marisa, but I did drop off a post-surgery care package filled with a few goodies I hoped my pal would enjoy—homemade peanut butter cookies, a couple magazines, and some packets of my favorite tea. A small but "active friend mode" gesture for an incredible person I want in my life for the long haul.

I also asked two of my DFNs, Anna and Jennifer, to play We're Not Really Strangers. They were excited to try, so we met at Anna's house for a Friendship and Ramen Night. (Nothing cryptic about the name of our soirée; we'd just been craving ramen.) As soon as we finished our bowls, we pulled out the game, read the instructions, and drew our first cards. Some have questions for your friends to answer about themselves, while others are designed to test their knowledge of you or your friendship.

One of the first cards we drew asked, "What do you want to make more time for? What's getting in the way of that?" Considering we're all working moms who had just spent the last half hour detailing how insane our lives were lately, we howled. We knew the answers to the second question, but hearing the answers to the first was fascinating. And there were more than a few surprises that night. Whenever someone answered a question, another woman would exclaim along the lines of, "Really? I wouldn't have thought that about you!" or "I never knew that!" or "I love that you remember that moment!"

After playing one round, meaning we worked our way through the game's three levels of questions, we called it quits. We agreed the game was amazing because we had fun learning new things about each other. Felt closer to each other. Wanted to play again soon.

And to close out Friendship and Ramen Night, I asked my girls what their friendship love languages are to make sure I'm showing my appreciation for them well. We had a fantastic discussion, and I floated home high on friendship vibes. The text messages the next day made my heart swell, too. Jen wrote, "Last night was so great" with a red heart emoji (I'm giving you the full visual here). Anna replied, "Wasn't it? I'm so grateful for you both," with a red heart emoji. And I said, "Same! I'm a lucky gal to have you both in my world," with a pink heart. Emoji hearts flying, love for each other clear. We give the intimacy game six thumbs up!

Next time I meet with them, and other DFNs in my life, I'll throw a few of those cards in my purse so we can keep getting to know each other better, even after all these years.

Historical Friends

After much inner turmoil over my longest-standing friendships, I feel some peace. I used to think our friendships have changed in adulthood because our lives have changed, but I recognize it's more than that: Our friendships are different because *we* are different. We're not the same people we were in our twenties, but who is? We have different interests, priorities, and life circumstances to navigate, which means I haven't been "doing life" with many of my old friends for a while. And accepting that I now have less in common with the crew, many of whom still see each other on the regular, takes away the sting I've felt over the distance between us.

Another thing that helps is giving myself the leeway to view our friendships as flexible, which means my forever friends *will* likely be in my life forever, just in a different way than before. And who knows? Maybe one day we'll move out of the ebb and into the flow. Regardless, I will always love them like family and want them in my life, however that looks.

Though I don't have the time or energy to see every one of my historical friends often, I am making the effort to see the ones I truly connect with, feel supported by, and share common interests with. I've initiated more coffee dates, planned lunches, gone on girls' trips, and organized couples' dinners to ensure we don't lose touch.

I even reached out to a friend I hadn't seen in more than eight years but was tight with for many years when we lived in the same city. For no reason other than distance (and, well, life's craziness), our friendship withered. But I have been missing her, so I recently sent her a message. Within minutes, she wrote me back, saying, "I literally was just saying I lost touch with you. Life gets busy and time seriously is going way too fast." After giving me a quick life update, she said, "I would LOVE to see you!" I was thrilled. We just had a catch-up over the phone and we're planning to meet in person soon. I can't wait.

But after everything I've tried and done the last few months, one of my biggest takeaways has been this: I can only control how I show up as a friend. Being the best version of myself I can for the people I love and cherish is my priority, so I'm going to give it my all.

I've also welcomed the idea that friendships can, and will, evolve. Some people will be in our lives forever, others might not. We need not beat ourselves up for needing to walk away or distance ourselves from friendships that aren't fulfilling, satisfying, or loving. But we should do everything we can to keep the ones that are.

Whether this chapter inspires you to better invest in your DFNs, reinvigorate friendships from the past, let go of those that aren't serving you, or seek new friends—or all the above—you've got this. Be positive, be consistent, be open.

And good friendships will follow.

THE CHEAT SHEET

- Conduct an audit of your friendships. Are they filled with positivity, consistency, and vulnerability? Are they supportive, fulfilling, and restoring? If so, cherish and protect those relationships. If not, don't be afraid to seek out new friendships.
- If you're looking to make new friends, pursue hobbies you enjoy, attend events you're interested in, and join clubs offering activities you love. Not only will you meet new

people who share similar interests, the consistent interaction will help establish your new friendships.

- Don't assume a friendship is over because it's in a low point. Friendships often ebb and flow. If you can view your relationships as flexible instead of fragile, you will sustain them better.
- Ask your friends, "What's your favorite way for me to show you how much I appreciate you?" Understanding their friendship love language will help you demonstrate your care and gratitude in ways that resonate with them.
- When your friends experience very high or low moments, that's your cue to kick into active friend mode. Take time to celebrate their wins and successes, and to support them through their losses and hard times.
- Be vulnerable with your friends. Share what's really going on in your world and how you're feeling. Giving your friends the raw, behind-the-scenes look at your life will build intimacy.
- Don't hide the time you spend with friends from your partner, kids, or family. Letting them see you prioritize friendships will teach your loved ones to do the same—and having that ability will benefit their health and well-being for the rest of their lives.
- To inspire deeper, different conversation with your friends, consider buying and playing the friendship edition of We're Not Really Strangers. You'll learn new things about each other, have fun, and strengthen your connection.
- Your number-one job as a friend is to ensure your friends leave your interactions feeling loved, supported, and uplifted. Bringing joy and positivity to your interactions will help your friendships flourish.

CHAPTER FIVE

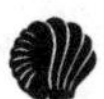

Make Peace with Your Body

When I was 12, I needed exploratory surgery. I had hurt my right knee during a wild tube ride behind a motorboat, and my leg refused to straighten afterward. My condition stumped my doctor, prompting him to book a knee arthroscopy. Shortly before I started seventh grade, I went to the hospital so a surgeon I'd never met could insert tiny cameras into my knee and look around.

I remember nothing about the experience except what the surgeon said when he entered my room. After one look at me resting in the hospital bed and a quick glance at my parents, he turned back to me and said, "They sure feed *you* well!"

Not to get too dramatic on you, but that moment is seared into my soul.

I was shocked, embarrassed, and ashamed. No one had ever made me feel bad about my weight before. And the craziest thing? I wasn't overweight or obese. Even if I were, what a jerk. I was just a girl going through puberty whose body was changing. How I wish I'd said something brilliant in reply to that doctor. Instead, I probably laughed off his hideous comment or said nothing. But I tucked his little jab away deep inside, as we all do when something stings.

Of course, I know you can relate to this story. You likely have similar experiences seared into your souls. Women deal with appalling, unsolicited commentary about our bodies all the time. Being young does not shelter us from it, even at the hands of health professionals who should know better.

Despite the experience with my surgeon, my body image and I escaped relatively unscathed. I credit team sports. Once my knee healed from the non-essential tissue tear—the doctor was good for a diagnosis, at least—I joined my school volleyball and basketball teams. For six years, I learned how good it felt to sweat, move, and compete. Body confidence was the result. But I didn't have a label for it back then; I just felt good in my skin. Pictures from that time show my weight fluctuating with the seasons, but I never weighed myself. I didn't worry about what I was eating or how much, and I rarely thought about how my body looked.

Incredible to think about now. How lovely. How rare. How freeing.

And how fleeting.

At some point in my early twenties, I became acutely aware of my body, maybe because I became more acutely aware of others' bodies. For the first time, I was consistently working out at the gym, where I lifted weights and ran on the treadmill. Seeing the fit bodies around me was inspiring and motivating but also had the unfortunate side effect of making me evaluate my body in a way I'd never done before. I was exercising but not eating well, placing me on the higher end of the healthy weight range for my height. I know this because I'd started to weigh myself. I was plump, yes, but not overweight, just like when I was 12. The difference was, this time, *I* was shaming myself for being fed too well—and I had the motivation to do something about it.

Losing weight became a priority. Among other changes to my diet, I stopped buying muffins for breakfast on the way to my university classes, ate dressing-free salad for lunch most days, and nixed my weekly Skor Blizzard from Dairy Queen. Then I read that a celebrity, maybe Jennifer Lopez, didn't eat past 7 p.m.

I could do that, I thought. So, I did.

But then I started to move the cut-off earlier and earlier. For a handful of months, I stopped eating anything after 2 or 3 p.m. and went to bed hungry. I knew this was not healthy or sustainable behavior. I didn't care. My body was getting smaller, and my clothes felt looser. In my twisted logic, the reward trumped the sacrifice.

Thankfully, I managed to end my flirtation with disordered eating before things worsened. I'm embarrassed to admit it was because of a guy.

When I met a law student at a friend's party and he asked me out for dinner, I said yes. Then I realized that if I wanted to do ordinary things like go on a dinner date—and *eat* the food—I would have to change my mindset and my behavior. I gave myself a pep talk and ate dinner with my date, but I remember struggling for months afterward to find a new eating groove. Occasionally, I'd end up on a food binge and then restrict my intake for a day or two in remorse. Or I'd eat normally but push myself extra hard at the gym to compensate. Exercise became more punishment than pleasure.

But things changed again in my late twenties and early thirties. I don't know what to credit other than I grew up. I wanted to find a wellness routine I could love and sustain for the rest of my life. More than anything, I craved balance and being at peace with my body.

Around this time, I was lucky to learn more about how to pursue that kind of lifestyle in my role as a health and wellness columnist for my city's major newspaper. Every day, I read new studies, interviewed brilliant nutrition and physical-health experts, and had the opportunity to try their advice. I found joy and satisfaction in every workout because exercise was for a different reason: to see how fast my body could run a three-mile race, how many pull-ups I could build up to, and how much weight I could squat. With goals to become faster and fitter, not smaller, going to the gym felt fun.

My eating leveled out, too, and I established healthy and sustainable habits. Most importantly, they were enjoyable. Fueling my body with satisfying, nutrient-dense meals and snacks felt good. Eating to feel great was my goal, not restricting foods to lose weight.

And that's how I've been living since. I don't diet. I don't fast. I try to eat well but enjoy everything in moderation and listen to my hunger cues. As for working out, I exercise often but not as hard as I used to, and I take more rest days. (See chapter 1 for the details!) My body has responded well. I have energy, my weight is healthy, and I'm injury-free. Fitness-wise, I'm in the best shape of my life.

I would love to tell you, then, that I never critique my body and only have thoughts of self-love and total body acceptance. But I am human. I have moments when negative self-talk creeps in, when I think or voice criticisms about how I've eaten or what the number on my scale says. These are ridiculous things to worry about, especially because I am the first to acknowledge I live in a thin body. Logically I know my body is privileged, yet self-critical thoughts are there, simmering underneath the surface and ready to boil up at any time.

I'm ready to stop them from simmering.

As a woman in midlife focused on feeling great and aging well, I want to annihilate negative self-talk for good. Be nothing but grateful for my body and its ability to move me through the world. Stop the undercurrent that strives for perfection. I want that for me, my friends and family, and you.

We all deserve to be at peace with our bodies.

Why is doing that so hard?

To answer that question, I first spoke with Dr. Jennifer Gaudiani, a woman passionate about helping people navigate complicated relationships with food and their bodies. Jennifer is a certified eating disorder specialist supervisor and fellow at the Academy for Eating Disorders, as well as the founder of the

Gaudiani Clinic in Denver, which provides specialized outpatient treatment for people of all ages with eating disorders or disordered eating of any type. Before launching her clinic in 2016, Jennifer spent eight years running Denver Health's medical-stabilization unit for critically ill adults with anorexia and bulimia. With more than 40 percent of people admitted age 30 and over, and more than 30 percent of people 40 and over, many of her patients were adult women. All were very ill, but that's not what people often noticed. "My patients, some of whom were weeks away from death, would literally be stopped on the street by strangers saying, 'You look amazing! What do you do?'" says Jennifer. "So, this society is terribly sick."

An Important Note

If you are struggling with an eating disorder and live in the United States, please contact the National Eating Disorders Association (NEDA) at 1-800-931-2237 or visit NationalEatingDisorders.org.

For help if you live in Canada, please contact the National Eating Disorder Information Centre (NEDIC) at 1-866-633-4220 or visit nedic.ca.

And *that*, right there, highlights why accepting our bodies is so hard. This is a news flash to no one, but we live in a world that idolizes thinness seemingly above all else. Whether someone praises us for being thin or shames us for being big, we have all grown up bombarded with versions of the same message: Thinness is the goal. No wonder our inner voices have started to chime in along the way, pointing out our "flaws" and pushing us to strive for perfection.

"When we struggle with some imperfection, it's not because our bodies are at fault. It's because society has given us the relentless message that we are never enough and only if we as closely as possible approximate the ideal will we have the right to speak our words, to voice our dissent, and to advocate for what we want," Jennifer says. "This is not about individual bodies. It has nothing to do with whether we have stretch marks or lots of body fat or an awkwardly balanced proportion of features. This is about individuals coming to harm from a system of oppression that wants to silence us and make us feel bad about ourselves."

Not only does society idolize thinness, but, as Jennifer says, Western medical systems assume fatness is all about individual choice and willpower, that there is a simple equation of calories in and calories out that determines size, and that if people could just eat less and move more, they would be able to live in thin bodies and reap the benefits, medical, societal, and otherwise. That's how most doctors continue to think and advise patients, says Jennifer, but that thinking is not only wrong, it's harmful.

She points to a meta review of scientific studies examining weight loss versus increased fitness and physical activity for reducing health risks among the obese. Ultimately the findings showed that focusing on weight loss alone is largely ineffective, and focusing instead on helping people get fitter and stronger yields equal or better results. It also helps people avoid weight cycling—the harmful cycle between losing weight on a diet and gaining it back again.

One study showed people who weight-cycled the most had a 99 percent increased risk of heart attack and a 92 percent increased risk of stroke compared to those who weight-cycled the least. But weight cycling is the almost inevitable result of dieting because, biologically, dieting doesn't work. "Our brains are trained to protect our body weight and save us from starvation," Jennifer says. "If we lose weight, the brain goes into overtime trying to help us fix that dreadful problem. It's not willpower. It's biology."

Rather than tell people to eat less and move more, which is ineffective and worsens health outcomes, Jennifer imagines a world where doctors give everyone a different message from childhood. It goes like this:

"The way to best health is to nourish your body to satisfaction, avoiding nothing but what you're allergic to and your gut can't tolerate. If you nourish yourself without dieting and stay as active as your interest and ability allow, you will end up in the healthiest possible body there is, you will avoid ending up in a body that is meaningfully heavier than your genetics would have predicted, and you'll live a better quality of life."

I love that message. It's positive, peaceful, and so different from the one we hear. Since Jennifer shared it with me, I've repeated it to myself and my loved ones.

I hope you keep it in mind, too, because we won't likely be bombarded with that kind of body-positive advice anytime soon. Though we hear more about body inclusivity and positivity these days, we still have a long way to go as a society. For proof, look no further than the demand for Ozempic, a diabetes drug that celebrities and everyday people are now taking to lose weight.

So, I'm repeating it again for good measure: Society is the issue here, *not* our bodies. If we can accept that, we take the first step toward loving ourselves, because having awareness helps us "unhook from the matrix," as Jennifer says, and begin to unwind the messages we've internalized from media, friends, family, teammates, coaches, colleagues, and healthcare practitioners our entire lives. "Then we start being able to imagine a different world," she says, "a world in which we don't denigrate ourselves in any way."

Let's imagine the self-love, body acceptance, and freedom in that world for a minute. But we don't have to imagine. Each one of us can help make it a reality. As Jennifer suggests, if women everywhere can challenge themselves to do these two things, we will be off to an excellent start:

1. **We can bravely, radically decide to stop talking negatively about our bodies, denigrating our food, and**

being ashamed of having needs. No more talking about feeling guilty for eating too much chocolate last night, for example, or voicing shame for putting on a few pounds, or lamenting how you look in a bathing suit. Jennifer says, "It doesn't mean we run around being like, 'I'm perfect.' It just means we stop denigrating ourselves."

2. **If we struggle to stop putting ourselves down for our own benefit, let's do it for the sake of those around us.** Altruism inspires many women, says Jennifer, which means we're more inclined to change our behavior if someone else will benefit. (Another societal problem, she adds, but it's the reality.) Everyone around us hears and feels our words, so we must use them carefully. "When we put ourselves down, we are essentially contributing to an invisible but highly toxic pollutant that harms our friends, partners, and children," Jennifer says. "If we can stop talking negatively about our own bodies for the betterment of others, and incidentally we ourselves benefit, then something important could happen."

Hearing Jennifer's words made me feel all the things: enlightened, inspired, and motivated to change. I also felt ashamed. Learning about my role in creating change forced me to face the uncomfortable realization that I've contributed to the invisible but toxic pollutant too many times to count. With my close friends, I've mentioned feeling guilty for putting on a few pounds, eating too much chocolate the night before, or feeling bad about my body. At the very least, I've voiced discontent about my body when someone else has voiced theirs. I want to stop doing that for my sake and the benefit of everyone around me.

Since speaking with Jennifer, I've worked hard to stop saying negative things about my body when I'm with friends, family, and even colleagues, and I've become hyper-aware of how I speak about myself around my daughter. Not only have I stopped voicing anything critical when I'm with her, but I try to be extra vocal about body-positive thoughts. I talk about how amazing our bodies are. How lucky we are to live in bodies that let us move, play, swim. How lifting weights makes me feel strong and capable. I can't be sure all the body-positive talk is helping, but there are signs. The other day, she flexed her 5-year-old muscles, kissed her right bicep, and said, "Mommy, I'm strong!"

Helping her feel good about her body is helping me feel good about mine. Consistently voicing appreciation for my body leaves little room for self-criticism.

But I'll warn you of a side effect: Once you stop saying bad things about yourself out loud, you will start noticing how often other women put themselves down. Since my chat with Jennifer, I can't go a single day without hearing a woman apologize for her appearance, voice a comment about wanting to lose weight, or feel guilty for indulging in a food craving. I'm not passing judgment at all. That's how I've been talking about myself and interacting with other women for a long time. But the comments make me sad, especially when they come out of the mouths of the people I love.

I'm also never sure how to reply. Whereas I used to offer a disparaging comment of my own in solidarity, I try not to do that now. Sometimes I dispute what they're saying and give compliments. Other times I just listen. But I figured there had to be a better response. After many months of wondering exactly what to say when someone I love criticizes her body or her needs, I decided to reach out to Jennifer for advice. She emailed me back to share the response she uses when someone in her life is speaking badly about herself: "You know my feelings on negative self-talk. I love you and invite you not to say things like that about yourself, for your sake and for others."

Brilliant and kind—and perhaps better delivered by a world-renowned authority on these matters. For my part, I can't say everyone in my life knows my feelings on negative self-talk (which are new, to boot), nor would I feel totally comfortable delivering that message to some of my loved ones. But I've been mulling over a version that feels true to me while still capturing the essence, and I've landed on one that I like: "I love you and hope you'll stop saying things like that about yourself. You are incredible as you are."

And that's the thing. I truly believe all the women in my life are incredible as they are. I would never notice the things they criticize about themselves, and I appreciate them for the many qualities that make them who they are. Whenever I feel the urge to put myself down in their presence, I remind myself they love me in the same way—and voicing whatever insecurity I have hurts me and them.

Though I haven't been perfect at squashing negative comments about my body or my food, I have come a long way in the past year. I would love to live in a world where women never say a negative word about themselves, so I promise to focus on keeping my negative comments from polluting our shared atmosphere. That's something I can control, something we can all control and work toward. No doubt, our efforts will add up and start to improve our collective well-being.

As we work on not criticizing our bodies out loud, another question remains: How do we stop our brains from being critical in the first place?

That may be too tall an ask of any woman, but we can start by realizing we have control over the thoughts we let ourselves pursue, says Dr. Margo Maine, an award-winning clinical psychologist specializing in eating disorders. Among other accomplishments, she is a founder and former advisor of the National Eating Disorders Association, and she has written many books, including *Pursuing Perfection: Eating Disorders, Body Myths, and Women at Midlife and Beyond*. At her private practice in Connecticut, Margo also sees patients, many of whom are high-functioning women in midlife.

Every day she helps these women tune into—and shift—their inner dialogues. And tuning in is a critical first step for all of us, no matter where we are on our body-image journey.

"One of the most important things we need to do as women is recognize our self-talk. Ask yourself, 'What do I expect of myself every day? What do I say to myself? And what do I say to myself about my body?'" she says. "It's not that bad thoughts don't come in. They do. But you don't have to give them any time whatsoever."

To explain why not dwelling on self-critical thoughts is so important, Margo draws inspiration from a form of moving meditation she loves to practice. "There is a principle in Qi Gong: Where your mind goes, your energy follows," she says. "So as soon as you start feeling something negative, put a check on it."

Stopping our minds from traveling down negative roads not only protects our energy and saves us from having to pull ourselves back to a positive place but keeps our brains from developing neural behavioral pathways that make habits so sticky. Every time we do or think something, we create a neural pathway, says Margo, and when we repeat the action, the pathway deepens. "Things we do all the time, like brushing our teeth, get these big superhighways in our brain," Margo says. Likewise, the more we think badly about ourselves, the deeper and more entrenched those highways become. "So, you must be careful about what you think. Don't let your mind go down the critical road."

Well, that ship has sailed, you're thinking.

That's what I thought, too. I've spent years harboring sneaky, negative thoughts about my body, so those highways have been paved and are well traveled. What next? Can we put down new roads and change our thinking in midlife? "Absolutely! It's never too late," Margo says. "Carving new neural behavioral pathways in our brains is possible and we can do it, but not without hard work."

Don't worry. Margo has suggestions to help us tackle the work. Here are a few of the strategies she recommends for any woman looking to shift her thinking:

1. **Embrace the idea of good enough.** Margo is passionate about sharing these four words with women: You are good enough. It's a tough idea for many of us to accept, though. Not only is it a foreign message, but Margo says some women view embracing "good enough" as giving up, as if it's the opposite of perfection—and perfection is what we've been taught to seek. But let's decide to be done with the idea of perfect bodies, perfect lives, perfect anything, and start appreciating who we are right now. Margo says, "We need to start being happy with good enough."
2. **Every night, thank your body for three things it did that day.** Whether you thank your body for being able to go for a run, play with your kids, or sit upright and observe the world around you, Margo recommends we all take a few minutes every night to express gratitude for the incredible bodies we inhabit. And it can be as simple as thanking our bodies for doing three things. "Let's appreciate these bodies and everything they do for us."
3. **Take careful inventory of the people around you.** To do this, ask yourself: Who do I hang out with—and do they bring out the best in me? This is a big question but an important one to answer. Margo says many of her patients switch peer groups after realizing their friends constantly obsess over their bodies or their competitive sports clubs push them to extreme behaviors. You may not need to walk away from a whole friend group, but identifying negative influences in your life—be they people, media, influencers, whatever—and avoiding them as best as possible is a smart move. So is prioritizing relationships with women you admire. "Who are your heroes? And are they heroes because of their bodies or something else?" Margo says. Spoiler alert: It's not because of their bodies. "Think of the women in your life that give you strength, courage, and love. Be sure *those* are the people you hang out with."

I didn't wait a day to put Margo's tips to use. The night we spoke, I crawled into bed and thought about everything my body had done that day. I carried heavy grocery bags up our front steps, sweat through a twenty-minute Peloton spin class, stood on my feet for hours in the kitchen to prep and cook food for the week ahead, played with my kids and helped them bathe, and did many other things I take for granted every day. I thanked my body for doing it all and told it to rest well.

Focusing on gratitude for my body every night has done me good. How exactly? Unlike how I could track my progress with numbers when I was trying to add muscle mass or tell you how my skin visibly changed after I improved my skincare routine, reporting on how my thinking has shifted is trickier. I can't point to specific measurements or outputs to highlight my progress, but I can tell you I am starting to think differently, feel differently, look at my body differently. Thanking my body every night—sometimes just for being healthy and helping me move through the world—helps me focus on everything I am thankful for and release vain annoyances and worries.

If those negative thoughts creep in, as they sometimes do when I'm getting ready in the morning or just before bed, I stop myself from going there and recite the "I am good enough" mantra. Some days, if I'm feeling extra spicy, I'll top it off with a "Thank you, body, you're amazing!" for good measure. And I might even do a little naked dance in my bathroom. But most of the time saying "I am good enough" is, um, enough.

Taking inventory of who and what I surround myself with has led to a lot of reflection about who I admire and why, and what their energy brings to my life—and vice versa. For the most part, my life is filled with positive, uplifting friends and family that bring out the best in me. I don't need a major overhaul in that department. The people who I spend the most time with make me feel fantastic, and I hope they feel the same about me.

But my Instagram feed? That needed some work.

You might think the first thing I did was unfollow all the popular fashion and media accounts that often share images of rail-thin models and celebrities, but I haven't. And I don't plan to. Fashion brings me too much joy. I will always enjoy scrolling through photos of runway shows, reading about style trends, and seeing who wore what to the Oscars. Those accounts, for me, are a must.

I did, however, unfollow or mute a handful of people—some I knew, others I didn't—that triggered something in me, whether it was an unhealthy body comparison or some kind of anxiety. And I made a point to seek out and follow more body-positive advocates, as well as women who share age-positive thoughts and insights. Curating my feed so that I'm exposed to more uplifting messages boosts my mood and my outlook on life.

Social media is one of many environmental inputs often contributing to the belief that thinner is better, says Summer Innanen, a Vancouver-based body-image coach helping women live beyond the scale. She asks her clients and all of us to consider the many other inputs we face daily. For instance, do you weigh yourself every morning? Listen to podcasts about weight loss? Is your workplace running a weight-loss challenge? Do you use a measuring tape or a certain pair of jeans to measure and assess your body? Do the shows you watch feature only thin bodies? "All of these things impact the belief system we have that thinner is better and bigger is bad," says Summer, "and if we have that belief system, we're going to think our bodies aren't good enough and we need to be thinner."

But the good news is we need not be stuck with these negative inputs.

Summer suggests ditching your home scale, anything you use to measure your body, TV shows and media that objectify women, social media accounts with "perfect" bodies, and clothes that no longer fit you. She also recommends we all stop commenting on others' bodies and food intake because, even if we think we're sharing a compliment about someone's weight loss or their drive to exercise, we're upholding harmful diet culture and body hierarchies. As for that workplace weight-loss challenge? Consider speaking to human resources, she suggests, and letting them know it promotes disordered eating and harmful ideologies about weight and health.

"Getting rid of these inputs is the first step because then we can start to change," says Summer, "and we can add stuff into our lives that's going to uphold the other belief system, which is that all bodies are good. Your value is not in your body size."

Aside from making sure your closet is filled with clothes that fit you, Summer suggests adding social media accounts to your feed that show fat bodies, aging bodies, diverse bodies. This sounds like a small change, but its impact cannot be overstated. Summer says her clients often report that switching up who they follow on social media has created the most profound change in their lives. "Social media is a huge factor," Summer says. "If you're only looking at photos of Gwyneth Paltrow–type people, that will be your baseline for how you look at yourself and measure up."

To help adjust your baseline, here are ten of the many Instagram accounts Summer recommends to her clients (in addition to her own, @summerinnanen). These and many others are helping reinforce the belief that all bodies are worthy of respect:

@iamchrissyking

@fierce.fatty

@amapoundcake

@saucye_

@glitterandlazers

@thedietrebellion

@black.woman.blooming

@antidietfatty

@dr_chairbreaker

@ameeistalking

Getting rid of harmful inputs and filling your feed with body-positive accounts will help shift your mindset and shake up your belief system that thinner is better. Changing your belief system is doable at any age, says Summer, and she's seen many clients in midlife overcome their body-image issues. But getting there will require intentional thought and practice, especially if you've spent the better part of your life hating your body. Like Margo, Summer asks women to reflect on how we speak to ourselves every day. Ideally, it is with kindness. "We want to build an inner voice of self-compassion instead of an inner critic, but it's not something that just switches on," she says. "It's like a muscle. The more we speak to ourselves with self-compassion, the easier it becomes."

Building our self-compassion muscle takes time, says Summer, so here are three steps to take when your inner critic voices negative self-talk of any kind:

1. **Recognize that negative thoughts about your body are not your fault.** As Summer and our other experts have shared, we aren't born believing thinner is better. We have learned and internalized these thoughts because we live in a culture that idolizes thinness, encourages the pursuit of "perfection," and makes us feel like our bodies are less than ideal. "This is a cultural issue, a near universal condition for women in the world," Summer says. "You're not defective for having these thoughts, and we can change them."
2. **Start to create a level of separation from your negative thoughts.** Whenever a negative thought creeps in, be it about your body, weight, or appearance, redirect the thought to acknowledge its societal root. For example, instead of saying, "I hate my body," Summer suggests trying, "I hate that I live in a culture that makes me feel like my body is a problem." Or it could be as quick as acknowl-

edging, "There's that voice of diet culture," or "That's the voice of beauty culture," or whatever the case may be. Creating a level of separation from your negative thoughts puts you in a better place to respond, Summer says.

3. **Make space for the feelings your thoughts bring up.** Negative thoughts often make us feel ashamed, sad, and disappointed. Rather than trying to ignore or suppress those emotions, Summer suggests acknowledging them and then speaking to yourself with self-compassion. Here's an example of how that inner talk could go: "I feel ashamed and I'm having a really hard moment here, but I want to remember that people love me for who I am. I have so much to offer the world that has nothing to do with how I look." Learning to comfort ourselves through difficult emotions, rather than trying to silence or battle our inner critics, makes it easier to eventually shift our thinking altogether, Summer says.

When Summer shared her tips, I felt like I'd gained the concrete, actionable steps I needed to build upon Margo's advice to not let your mind go too far down the critical road. Because, as both women said, it's normal to still have negative thoughts even as we learn to treat ourselves with greater compassion. How we respond and speak to ourselves in those moments is what matters.

Since speaking with Summer, I've been shifting any negative thoughts about myself to account for where they come from. For example, when I wasn't thrilled recently to see I'd gained a few pounds (more on that in a second), I said, "There's the voice of diet culture!" and reminded myself my value has nothing to do with my weight. And I can attest that the more I practice these steps and speak to myself with self-compassion, the less awkward it feels. My inner voice is slowly shifting. She is kinder, more accepting, and less concerned about having me step on a scale.

But I must be honest, as I was with Summer when we spoke: My daily weigh-in would be a hard habit to break. For the sake of my fitness chapter, I got used to weighing myself daily to track changes in muscle and weight, although my goal was never to lose weight during that experiment. Now that it's over, I'm still curious about my muscle, but I *could* stop weighing myself—and Summer thinks I should, as should every woman, because we tend to let the number on the scale dictate how we feel about ourselves. "Stepping on a scale is not a behavior of self-compassion. It is not reinforcing that you are good enough just as you are," she says. "You want to take actions that align to the belief system we want to have. I would highly encourage you to get rid of the scale."

At the very least, she encouraged me to pay attention to how I feel before I step on the scale. Anxious? Looking for validation? She says there are underlying reasons women weigh themselves and, in many cases, it comes down to wanting a sense of control or validation.

I don't know about you, but both ring true to me. I've come a long way in my thinking, but the 12-year-old, body-shamed girl inside me wants to monitor and control my weight, to applaud when my weight stays in a range that seems "good," whatever that is. But placing all the blame on that girl would be a cop-out. I'm 44 as I write this and, while I'm not trying to lose weight, I'm also not thrilled when I gain weight.

As a woman who considers herself pretty body positive, I feel shameful even sharing that, but I hope you understand.

Thankfully, Summer does.

In one of her newsletters (which I highly recommend you sign up for at summerinnanen.com), she discussed how most of us are in a tug-of-war between two paradigms—one that has conditioned us to believe our bodies are a problem and weight loss is the solution, and one that is encouraging us to be body positive and accept our bodies. "We can't simply pull the cord away from diet culture and expect to never feel drawn back again," she wrote. "It is normal to hold two perspectives that conflict with one another. You can have compassion for yourself for wanting to lose weight, while wanting to accept your body."

Body acceptance grows, she says, when we question and challenge why we feel the way we do and refuse to engage in the behaviors that uphold the thin ideal.

Thanks to the experts' advice, I've made strides on that front. Obviously, I have some to go. I'll keep striving to align my thoughts and behaviors with the belief I want to have now and always—that I am good enough, no matter what. It's a complicated endeavor, but I will remind myself I don't need to be perfect. My body doesn't need to be perfect. And learning to accept my body doesn't mean I have to love my body.

If that last line surprised you, you're not alone.

When I started writing this chapter, I was on a mission to determine how we can learn to love our bodies. I even tentatively titled it "Love Your Bod. Love Yourself." I was as surprised as you to find out that loving our bods shouldn't be the goal.

Not even close.

"You don't have to love your body. I just want people to not care so much about it, to know they're good enough regardless of how their body looks," Summer says. "Asking women to love our bodies almost does a disservice because it's another expectation we have to live up to. I want you to get to a place where you feel neutral in your body, where you can look in the mirror, like what you see or not, but be able to go on with your day and feel good about yourself. That's a freeing place to be."

When Summer shared her take, I felt my inner axis shift, my thinking change. I still get shivers thinking about the moment she blew my mind. Why? Because the idea of working toward feeling neutral in my body, in *our* bodies, is such a liberating thought. We have enough goals we set for ourselves, enough ideals and standards we hold ourselves up against. Let's forget about needing to love our bodies!

The idea of becoming body neutral—comfortable enough in my skin to get on with my life and not really think about my body—makes my soul feel good. It also feels like a more realistic, peaceful way to think about my body image as I age. I know my body will change in many ways if I'm lucky enough to grow old, and being body neutral will serve me well.

Aiming for body neutrality doesn't mean we shouldn't treat ourselves with love, speak to ourselves with love, or comfort ourselves through hard moments with love. It just means we should take the pressure off loving our bodies. They are good enough as they are.

We are good enough as we are. Yes, YOU! You are good enough. Never forget it.

THE CHEAT SHEET

- Nix the idea of perfection and embrace the idea of being good enough.
- Be kind to yourself. When a negative thought creeps in, remind yourself it's not your fault, create a level of separation by acknowledging the voice you're actually hearing, and speak to yourself with compassion about your true worth, which has nothing to do with how you look.
- Remove inputs in your life contributing to the belief that thinner is better. Curate your Instagram feed, stop weighing yourself every day, get rid of clothes that are too small. In their place, follow social media accounts featuring diverse bodies, abilities, and ages, and buy clothes that fit you.
- Stop voicing criticisms aloud about your body, appearance, and needs. If you can't stop for yourself, do it for the sake of those around you.

- Ditch the diets. They don't work and they're harmful. Trust that if you nourish to satisfaction and move your body regularly, your health will thrive.
- Every night before bed, thank your body for three things it did that day. No matter our size, insecurities, or self-criticisms, our bodies are glorious. Let's give them the props they deserve.
- Don't worry about trying to *love* your body. Instead, aim for body neutrality. Being able look at yourself in the mirror, like what you see or not, and continue to enjoy your day is a freeing way to live.

CHAPTER SIX

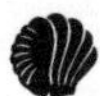

Stoke Your Creative Fire

I WRITE FOR A LIVING BUT DO NOT CONSIDER MYSELF PARTICULARLY creative.

Aside from the countless magazine and newspaper articles I've written, the press releases and websites I've composed for my communications clients, and the books I've ghostwritten, I haven't turned a single innovative idea into something I could share with the world. Nor have I produced any original ideas or objects.

(Wait, does producing humans count? If so, I was a creative genius in 2016 and 2018.)

My life is hectic, demanding, and messy, and it doesn't leave much room for getting creative just for the sake of it. I'm guessing many of you are in the same situation. We're too busy working, seeing friends, raising kids, traveling, folding laundry, squeezing in a quickie with our partners as said kids watch TV shows on Saturday afternoons (just me?), and doing all the other life stuff.

But as a kid, I used to love writing poems, creating dance routines with my friends, and drafting short novels I would force my babysitters to read. And when my French grandmother, my beloved mémère, taught me to sew, knit, and crochet in my teens, I went through a lengthy period of creating ill-advised and, honestly, ill-formed garments, like jeans with panels of colorful fabric I'd sew down the sides of the legs.

Even in my twenties, I created for fun. While studying journalism in Toronto, I wrote song lyrics and dreamed up a bare-bones storyline for an Aerosmith musical. I mean, it practically writes itself. "Janie's Got a Gun." "Cryin.'" "I Don't Want to Miss a Thing." Why has no one written this musical?!

Now, in my early forties, it feels like my creative juices have evaporated. Poof. Gone.

But I refuse to believe they're gone for good. Because, though I'm happy to ditch those old jeans, getting creative is something I miss.

Many women I know feel the same way.

"I have a thirst for creativity, things like painting and cross-stitching. It makes me feel freer and more connected to who I am, not just a mother, wife, employee," said Sarah, a community investment and public affairs administrator with one of my corporate communications clients. As important as creating is to her, the daily grind makes it hard to carve out space for those practices. "I get pulled into new creative outlets, but then life happens, and they fall away. We live in a world that's so focused on productivity and results at work and at home. Taking time for ourselves feels selfish."

Alicea, a colleague of hers, can relate. With three kids, a full-time job in finance, and an active social life, she has little time to dig into creative endeavors she used to enjoy, like baking, DIY projects, and sewing.

Scratch that. She has *no* time.

"I've prioritized other things and let those creative outlets go. But am I prioritizing what I need or what other people need?" she said. "Creativity continually falls to the bottom of the list."

No matter our careers or life circumstances, many women feel like taking time to pursue creative outlets—activities that bring us joy, delight us, engage us—is a frivolous endeavor at best, selfish at worst.

Rest assured, ours is not a new plight. And Brigid Schulte wants to make sure all women know that.

"Women have never had a history or culture of leisure or play throughout all of human history," Brigid told me over Google Meet one day from her home in Virginia, Alexandria. She is a Pulitzer Prize–winning journalist, author of the *New York Times* bestseller *Overwhelmed: Work, Love and Play When No One Has the Time,* and director of the Better Life Lab, the work-family justice program at New America. "Leisure time was afforded to the upper classes, usually men of privilege, and the drudge work was left to all the servants, slaves, and women. We've made a lot of progress in recent decades, but there's still a lot of baggage."

There's a lingering undercurrent that there is something unseemly about a woman who is not busy, Brigid says. There's also a weird stigma that women who take unstructured and undefined time to themselves are selfish, because we have been raised to believe our highest and best value is to care for other people. Caring for others is beautiful and valuable, of course. "But you know what? Men need to take time to care as well, not just women," Brigid says. "Caring is a human quality. And women also need to take care of themselves, to put themselves into the equation."

Doing that means making space for our creative outlets, whims, urges. Whatever our hearts desire and our souls need.

"Creativity is critical for being human, just to have time and space that isn't tied to your to-do list, to doing or being productive," Brigid says. And though people often associate creativity with activities like painting or dancing, to her, it's more about creating the space to be open to receive whatever inclination comes. If you feel like doing any of those activities, fantastic. But creativity can also be more nuanced, less structured. You might feel like walking around the block or playing in your backyard. Anything is valid.

"See what comes to you," Brigid says. "What do you feel like doing in that moment? What do you need? And if you don't know, it's probably because we're so busy."

To help us tune into what we need and make space for it in our lives, Brigid recommends the following:

1. **Pause.** "Just stop, sit, and breathe," Brigid says. Allow yourself to think about what would be fun and be open to receiving whatever comes. There are no bad ideas.
2. **Prioritize fun.** Once you figure out what you want to try, make a plan. If you love ticking things off a to-do list, add your activity to it, suggests Brigid. You can also book time off in your calendar. "And if you can't make it at that time, move it somewhere else," she says. "That way it's like you're keeping a promise to yourself."
3. **Recognize the external pressures you face.** For millennia, women have been expected to be industrious, work hard from sunup till sundown, care for others before caring for themselves. "Those pressures aren't just external," Brigid says. "You have internalized them, so they appear as little voices in your head." Those little voices often dismiss our creative wants and needs as silly or unproductive or make us feel we haven't earned the time to engage in them. "But ask yourself, whose voice is telling me that? Turn the volume on it down, and listen to your intuition, your gut, your soul."
4. **Give yourself permission to have fun.** No matter what you want to do—play the guitar, experiment with makeup, learn to canoe—recognize it's a valuable use of your time and make space for it. You don't need to justify your creative pursuit, least of all to yourself. Brigid says, "Once you give yourself permission, that creates energy, goodness and positivity, and a better understanding of how you need to incorporate that activity into your life."
5. **Aim for creative pulses.** Brigid says people usually associate creativity with getting into a flow state, the magical zone when you're fully immersed and engaged in a creative

practice over a long, concentrated time. But you don't have to spend all day on your activity. Instead, try incorporating small chunks of fun into your day. Brigid leads by example. When writing a book, as when we spoke, she sets a timer for thirty minutes of work and then breaks for a creative pulse. "As crazy as this sounds, I have a jigsaw puzzle on my dining room table right now, and it's so motivating. I give myself ten minutes to work on it, and then get back to work," she says. Building short, creative breaks into your schedule adds fun to your day and keeps your mind fresh. "The brain can do anything if it knows a break is coming."

6. **Find like-minded peers.** "If you're going to make time and space for creativity, that's an act of resistance. You're a rebel against the overworked culture," says Brigid. It's hard to fight the status quo alone, so find peers, friends, or online groups who, like you, are on a journey toward more creativity and can support you on yours.

7. **Pay it forward.** Brigid has seen many women pull up the drawbridge after themselves, voicing comments like, "I didn't get childcare when I needed it, so why should you?" Don't be a queen bee like that. Mentor someone younger than you, be part of the change, and help make life better for other women. "Tap into generosity and gratitude, and pay it forward," she says, "and recognize that this is bigger than you."

Brigid's words hit deep.

I love my hectic, demanding, and messy life, but I've been missing a creative outlet, something just for me and my soul. Until recently, I didn't even know what I wanted or needed to fill that void.

And until speaking with Brigid, I didn't appreciate how creativity (and our ability to access it) is political. But it makes total sense. To be creative, we need time, and society would have women spend our time elsewhere—on our families, at work, on drudge work. Even when no one speaks those words aloud, our inner voices pipe in to give us the message. Shunning our to-do lists in favor of activities that interest us, make us happy, and feed our souls does feel like an act of rebellion.

I'm here for the uprising.

And so is Jill Margo, a creative nonfiction writer and pressed flora artist based in Victoria, British Columbia.

"Time is a feminist issue. We are in a culture where time is power, and who owns the most time? White cis-gendered men, generally speaking," she told me while chatting over Google Meet. "How much free time you have depends on your social and economic status, so as a global majority, women have less time."

Jill is passionate about helping people the most impacted by patriarchy and other forms of oppression live better, more fulfilled lives through creative practices that feel generative, sustainable, and liberatory. She created a program called The Creative Good to do just that, so I reached out to glean her tips for experienced creators and newbies alike.

Like Brigid, she says recognizing that the issues women face are societal, not personal, is vital when looking to spark creative practices. On her website, thecreativegood.ca, she describes how we've internalized those external pressures—and how they interfere with our ability to create: "Worried about using your voice and taking up space? Thank you, patriarchy and white supremacy! Think you're too old and it's too late? Thank you, ageism! Think you're failing because you're too exhausted from your job to make art? Capitalism, I'm looking at you!"

The point? Feelings that hold us back from getting creative are *not* personal failings. They stem from collective issues, and Jill helps women and everyone she works with shake off those restrictive thoughts to use their voices, create art, and "shine their damn lights anyway."

There's too much at stake for our well-being not to.

"Creativity is a form of self-care, and to me, self-care is anything that helps us come home to ourselves," she says. (Such a beautiful thought, no?) And because we are all unique beings, our creative interests will be, too. Jill loves to turn pressed flowers from her garden into artwork. Some of her clients work on visual journals. Others paint, write, or make music. No matter the outlet, she says creative practices help us be in deeper relationships with ourselves. "It's part of our humanity to create."

If you're unsure how to start creating, Jill has thoughts.

When you have an idea for a creative project—heck, even the glimmer of an idea—don't feel you have to go all in or invest major time or money. Jill recommends a discovery phase first when you find small, simple, and affordable ways to explore your creative activity. Curious about painting? Buy a cheap watercolor set. Interested in a textiles project? Mess around with fabrics you find around your house. "Just start playing and see what that leads to."

And no matter where you are in your creative process, give yourself permission to make bad stuff. Seriously. Whatever you make does *not* have to be beautiful. There are way more important reasons to create, Jill says. "Do you enjoy the process? Is it delightful? Does it make you feel good? That's what counts."

Also, she says anyone who wants more creativity should start taking in more creativity: Read good books. Look at paintings. Listen to new music. "Output depends on input, so look for what you like and fill your well."

But inspiration will only get us so far.

Once we've played, experimented, and landed on a creative project to tackle or practice to engage in, we need productive habits to get it done, Jill says. Lucky us, she has some to share. She calls them The Three Good Habits, which apply whether you're a creative newbie or an experienced pro.

The beauty of her system is it will accommodate fluctuations in your capacity while keeping your creative spirit alive, an important consideration for Jill and her clients. "I came up with this system as a person with chronic illness because I can vary wildly in my capacity," she says. "This will work whether you want to create as a form of self-care and for your own edification or you want to do this as a career."

Without further ado, here are The Three Good Habits for anyone who wants to create:

1. **Make art for fifteen minutes a day, most days.** Some might think spending fifteen minutes on something creative is insignificant, but it has cumulative impacts. You could even have a "micro-practice" and create for only fifteen minutes weekly. "The secret of the 15s is that they're not really about the art you make," Jill says. "It's about having a container for art making, training yourself to consistently show up and hold that container open."
2. **Prioritize three small and strategic weekly tasks.** At the start of every week, assess your schedule and aim to complete three realistic things. Jill calls this setting "triorities," which can be as simple as tidying your creative space, drawing a sketch, or finishing a draft chapter of the book you're working on. Accomplishing small tasks related to your project will maintain your momentum.
3. **Review your progress and plan regularly.** Jill and her clients review their progress every week, month, and season, which helps people find patterns throughout the year and plan for the seasons ahead. Setting goals by season instead of at the start of every calendar year is a more intuitive, forgiving way to operate. "We're not machines designed for seasonless productivity. We need to allow ourselves to have ebbs and flows, to readjust our rhythms every few months," she says. "When you're working seasonally, it's short enough to not lose sight of your goals but long enough to get things done."

Armed with Jill's and Brigid's incredible insights and advice, I was excited to tune into my innermost wants and needs. Stoke my creative fire. Create something ugly. (Given my history with the jeans and all.)

But where to begin? I had zero contenders for creative outlets, so I took Brigid's advice. I paused one Sunday morning. I sat down. I breathed. Nothing came to me other than the urge to tidy my living room. But I didn't.

Down with the patriarchy! Screw drudge work!

Who are we kidding? I tidied it later that day. (But also, my husband is an incredibly helpful, hardworking partner who more than upholds his share of the household drudge work. Thank you, Cam.)

I didn't feel a creative spark that day or the next few days, but my subconscious wheels had been set in motion. I had created the space to let creativity in and that was enough because the answer finally came to me: knitting! I would learn to knit again!

Just thinking about picking up those needles stirred something in my soul.

It had been decades since my grandmother taught me the basic stitch, but I remember savoring the knitting process. Feeling joy in using my hands and creating something tangible. Reveling in the quiet afternoons sitting by her side, her demeanor patient and calm as she fixed my mistakes. My grandmother passed away in 2018. Knitting, I knew, would make me feel like coming home to myself and her.

I couldn't wait to get going. After some quick online research, I signed up for an affordable three-week knitting class for beginners at a studio near our house. Here's a peek into what happened during my creative discovery phase:

Week 1

I showed up to my first class feeling excited but nervous, envisioning a room full of women better knitters than me, like an army of knitting wizards lying in wait. But there was only one other student there, a woman my age, and our instructor, a man named Paul who runs bike programs for kids and teaches knitting on the side.

We started with the basics. Paul taught us to cast yarn onto needles, perform knit and purl stitches, and read a pattern. We put our newfound skills to work, each starting a scarf to work on over the coming weeks.

Work on it I did. I incorporated a few fifteen-minute creative pulses every day, knitting at night while the kids watched TV and during workdays at home when I'd break to stitch a few rows before returning to work. Over the weekend, I knit for longer chunks of time as the kids played nearby. And Jill was right: Fifteen-minute creative work periods start to add up and make a difference.

By the end of week 1, I was hooked (apologies for the needlework joke).

Week 2

I was so excited to work toward a finished product—my first ever—that I brought my project on a flight to Toronto. In constant fear I would drop stitches or have some other kind of knitting emergency, I pictured having to stand up and ask, "Is there a knitter on the plane?" Thankfully, I had no such issue.

But I had plenty of screw-ups, one of which forced me to rip out many rows and start again. What's wild: I loved the process so much that I didn't even mind. (I may have uttered a choice word or two.) I didn't let *every* mistake derail my progress, though. Knitting is, without a doubt, teaching the perfectionist in me to let go and not care so much about mistakes. Besides, and as Paul sagely pointed out, "There's a lot of fudging things in knitting." I'm learning to accept and work with imperfections, a skill that will serve me beyond my creative outlet. And I'm embracing a philosophy Brigid shared when we chatted: "Done is better than perfect."

By the end of week 2, my camel-colored scarf was well underway.

Week 3

At the start of our third and final class, I showed Paul my work, feeling good about how far I'd come. Then my fellow student showed up, opened her bag, and unfurled a fully finished scarf with nary a flaw.

I knew it—knitting wizard.

Whatever. I had to remind myself this was about *my* creative journey. I had rediscovered an activity I loved and already had my sights set on my next project: a chunky, oversized, colorful cardigan. "The way to improve is to challenge yourself," Paul had told us. Knitting a sweater would fit the bill, I thought. Before class finished, he reviewed my sweater pattern, gave me some tips, and wished us both well on our future projects. And as we left the studio that day, he turned to the other student and said, "I've never, in the history of this class, had someone finish the whole scarf by the end of week three!"

Thank you, Paul. Hearing that meant more to me than you will ever know.

Considering I finished my scarf shortly after and immediately started my next project, my discovery phase was a massive success.

Since then, I've knitted two chunky, pastel sweaters with beautiful wool from a European company called We Are Knitters, attended a knitting night at the studio in search of like-minded peers, and half-finished my first knit dress. I also recently started setting feasible triorities; this week I want to find a sweater pattern for my kids, organize the needles and yarn I'm amassing, and finish the back panel of my dress. In fact, excuse me as I pause for a fifteen-minute break to knit a few rows.

Okay, I'm back.

Weaving creative pulses throughout my day—usually fifteen to twenty minutes long, per the experts' tips—has made a significant difference in my life, somehow rounding out and softening my days. I could lose myself in the process for hours if given the chance. The fact that I end up with wearable pieces at the end is a bonus. (And, gals, they're way cuter than my sewn jeans!)

The advice I've incorporated has stoked my creative fire and, importantly, empowered me to take the time I need to keep it burning bright. Carving out space from my hectic life for fun and leisure isn't selfish. It's necessary. My life feels fuller than before, as does my creative well. Maybe one day I'll learn to crochet again or take a macrame class to make wall hangings, a hobby my great-grandfather pursued many years ago. I'm open to receiving whatever comes.

For now, though, I'm set. And I'm grateful.

Knitting makes me feel like I'm coming home to myself. I feel at peace, happy, and calm. And I'm reminded of the love and support my mémère gave me all those years ago. I miss her all the time, and knitting makes me feel closer to her and the woman I want to become.

Which creative activity would make you feel the same?

No matter what piques your interest, I hope you grant yourself permission to explore the idea and invest your time. Stoke that creative fire, babe, because it sure feels good.

Let's shine our damn lights together and create.

THE CHEAT SHEET

- Recognize that voices in your head seeking to dampen your creativity are not yours; they are external messages we have all internalized. Choose to turn the volume on them down, listen to your gut, and tune into what you need.
- Take a pause from the demands of daily life to sit and breathe. Reflect on what you feel like doing, anything that could bring you joy, fun, and delight. Be open to receiving whatever idea comes.
- When you feel a creative spark, conduct a discovery phase. Find small, affordable ways to explore what your creative

practice could be, turn into, and entail. Most importantly, have fun.

- Infuse short, creative pulses into your day, most days. Spending ten to fifteen minutes on something creative—even only once a week—is motivating and maintains momentum on whatever creative project you're tackling.
- Plan your creative breaks. Add them to your to-do list and block time off in your calendar. If that time doesn't work, reschedule instead of canceling.
- At the start of every week, prioritize three small, strategic tasks related to your project or craft. Review your progress at the end of each week, month, and season. Understanding your patterns will help you set realistic goals for the seasons ahead.
- If you want more creativity, start taking in more creativity. Go to art galleries, read more books, and listen to music. It can be hard to create from an empty well, so fill yours.

CHAPTER SEVEN

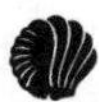

Tame Your Bad Habits Without Giving Them Up for Good

I LIKE TO DRINK WINE.

Sue me.

It's not that I'm proud of having a wine habit. But I have so few vices in my life that I have desperately clung to the belief that I should be allowed this one, right?

RIGHT?!

Not quite, says almost anyone who knows about this stuff.

By "anyone," I mean world-renowned experts and institutions. And by "stuff" I mean what it means to treat our bodies well, feel good every day, and live a long time. Because the evidence is in, my friends—has been for a long time, actually—and if you haven't heard, alcohol isn't good for us.

A quick and depressing overview: In a World Cancer Research Fund landmark study published in 2007 called "Food, Nutrition, Physical Activity, and the Prevention of Cancer," a key finding was that alcohol, a carcinogen, is a cause of cancer. Ideally, the study said, we would avoid alcohol completely. The recommendation tracks with Canada's Guidance on Alcohol and Health, newly revamped guidelines issued in early 2023 that warned no amount of alcohol is safe to consume (!). To minimize the risks associated with drinking—several types of cancer, heart disease, and stroke, to name a few—they suggested everyone consume no more than two drinks per week. (Cue mass disbelief, outrage, and sadness across Canada.)

Guidelines in the United States remain more lenient; women should consume no more than seven alcoholic drinks per week, and men should consume no more than fourteen. Still, the Centers for Disease Control and Prevention advise: "Drinking less is better for health than drinking more."

I can't argue with that logic. Accepting it deep in my soul, however, sucks. Really and truly sucks, especially because I love everything about wine.

I love learning about it, tasting different varietals, discovering something new, and noticing how my preferences shift as I age. I love sharing a bottle of rosé with friends, preferably while sitting on a patio in the summer. I love ordering a special bottle when dining out with my husband, Cam, to celebrate good news. I love drinking Chablis with a home-cooked meal. From the moment we uncork a bottle to when we savor the last drop, I love it all.

Have I mentioned I'm into wine?

But lest you think I'm only into vino, you should know there are many spirits that float my booze-loving boat. Margaritas, Champagne, gin and tonics, mimosas, and—sometimes, just sometimes when I'm feeling wild—Baileys in my coffee on vacation. It sounds like a lot, but I haven't been drinking them all at once, people! And I haven't been drinking every day. It's fair to say that, for most of my adult life, I have been a social drinker, picking and choosing my spots to have an alcoholic beverage or two or seven.

Things changed over the pandemic, though.

Like many people, my hubby and I developed a drinking habit while cooped up at home. Happy hour went from being an occasional treat on the weekend to a nearly everyday occurrence. We would pour a gin and tonic at 4 p.m. on a Tuesday to celebrate having quasi-successfully juggled working from home with keeping our kids entertained, shake up a margarita on a Thursday to make things seem more festive when we hadn't left the house for days, and have wine whenever we made a yummy dinner. And because we had lots of time to cook at home, yummy dinners were the norm.

When the pandemic ended and the lockdown rules disappeared, one thing stuck around: the urge to have happy hour on the regular. And though I wasn't particularly worried about my alcohol intake, I also am no fool. There's no dismissing the evidence that alcohol is detrimental to us in many ways, nor do I love the blah, groggy feeling that lingers the day after having a few drinks—a feeling that's only getting worse with age. I realized, too, that drinking less would be good not only for me but for our kids. As they get older and pay more attention to how we eat and drink, I want to be the best role model I can.

So, after a few discussions about alcohol and the too-prominent role it had been playing in our lives, Cam and I agreed to tame the habit we'd established. We aimed to drink less without giving it up for good. We said we'd try. We *did* try.

But I regret to inform you: Breaking bad habits is hard.

Preaching to the choir, you say. The big, habit-laden choir. Because I'm sure that if you've ever tried to imbibe less, curb your online shopping habit (same), quit digging into the Costco-sized bag of kettle-corn-flavored PopCorners when you're anxious (just me?), limit the time you spend scrolling social media (who hasn't?), or get any unwelcome habit under control, you know what it's like to try.

And you probably know how it feels to fail.

That's because habits are sticky. They don't want to be broken. They don't want to die. They want, my friends, to live forever. Why? Because they think they're doing us a favor.

"Habits are a design feature of the brain. The way that brains are built, they assume that when you develop a habit, that's the way thing are always going to be," says Dr. Russell Poldrack, a psychologist, cognitive neuroscientist, professor of psychology at Stanford University, and the author of *Hard to Break: Why Our Brains Make Habits Stick*.

This design feature is handy for most things in our lives, says Russell, because it allows us to accomplish routine tasks without much thought. To illustrate: If we had to decide how to brush our teeth, brew our coffee, make breakfast, and drive to work, we'd be mentally exhausted every day by 9 a.m. Many habits developed out of repetition are our friend because they let us move through the world with ease and little cognitive effort.

But as we can agree, not all habits are good for us. And in a cruel twist, they're often the ones that develop when we experience pleasurable, enjoyable, or good events that trigger our brains' reward centers (think: winning a hand of blackjack or sharing a social media post that gets tons of love). What makes these pleasure-based habits so sticky is the presence of dopamine, the feel-good neurotransmitter that can lead us to develop unhelpful, even harmful, habits.

Dopamine is fundamental to building habits, says Russell, because it tells the brain whether the world is better or worse than we expected and, here's the rub, primes the brain to act accordingly in the future. As he explained in a 2021 article for Princeton University Press, "When we take an action that leads to an outcome that is better than we expected, a little squirt of dopamine gets sent to the habit system. This causes the connections between the neurons that produced the behavior to become stronger, so the next time we are in the same situation, we are more likely to take the same action."

Dopamine is the major difference between the habits that help you breeze through your day and the ones you'd like to shake. Highly rewarding substances—or the ones our brains deem rewarding, at least—hijack our habit-making system so that not only do we want to consume them when they're available, but we crave them and seek them out when they're not. "When you have a habit that's related to highly rewarding substances like food, drugs, or alcohol, it's different than the habit of where you turn when you're driving to work because it engages what we call emotional systems," Russell says. "We don't feel a craving to turn right at the intersection, but we do feel a craving to have happy hour or that glass of wine."

We do, Russell. We sure do.

You know what else I crave and seek out? My Instagram feed.

Most of us can relate to feeling the itch to pull out our phones and check our feeds, and that's because using social media creates those giddy dopamine squirts. Anytime we get a like on a photo or post, a retweet, or any notification, dopamine is released, creating the feel-good, reward stimulation in our brains, setting us up to crave more hits in the future, and encouraging us to seek them out.

So, no matter the habit or vice you're wrestling with, be it wanting to cut down the time you spend on social media, stop reaching for chips when you're stressed, quit consuming excessive sugar, or curb the urge to have a regular happy hour, the point is a habit is a habit is a habit. And though your brain wants to keep your habits ready and willing to jump into action on your behalf, change is possible at this stage of life. Hard, but doable. "It's always hard, regardless of how old you are, but it's certainly not impossible at any age," Russell says. "There are a lot of good examples of people who have made significant changes later in life and been successful at it."

All we need is some time, forethought, and practice. As for willpower? It doesn't play the role you probably think. Russell says research suggests people with higher self-control don't suppress more momentary urges than those with poor self-control. But self-control *can* help us avoid situations that trigger our urges or habits, a critical piece when breaking bad habits.

Because once a habit is triggered, it's incredibly hard to stop it. Despite your best, logical intentions, the prefrontal cortex, which is responsible for things like reasoning and impulse control, ultimately gets outgunned by your brain's reward and motivation systems, says Russell. That's why your number-one strategy for breaking a habit is to stop it from being triggered in the first place. Here are some tips on how to do that—and what to do when you can't:

1. **Figure out the triggers for your habit and try to remove them from your life.** Identify the things that kickstart your habit, be it seeing ice cream in the freezer, wanting to smoke whenever you go to a bar, feeling stressed, or driving past a casino every day on your way home from work. "Get those triggers out of your life as much as you can," Russell says. Some fixes will be more doable than others. You can stop buying ice cream, meet your friends at a coffee shop instead of a bar, have a bath or meditate when stressed, take a new route home. Since avoiding triggers is critical to defeating the habits they cue, eliminating things from your life that drive you to your habit will have a big impact. But life is complex and that's not always a feasible strategy, especially if your trigger is an emotion, a place you frequent often, or even a person. Russell says, "Sometimes you can't avoid your trigger, like if it's your partner." (Yep, that would be a tough one.) For situations when you can't eliminate or avoid your trigger, proceed to step 2.
2. **If you can't remove the trigger from your life, have a strategy for when you face it.** If your goal is to not eat ice cream at 7 p.m., it's easy to tell yourself that when you wake up in the morning. But when 7 p.m. rolls around and the craving hits, what will your strategy be? It's worth planning out—and planning in detail, while you're at it. In psychology, this type of plan is called an "implementation intention," says Russell, because it details how you intend to implement

your goals when you're faced with your trigger. "It's easy to have the goal when the habit is not right there," he says. "When the glass of wine is right in front of you, it's a lot harder to make sure that your goal gets engaged." (Truth.) Here's what helps: making the intention as specific as possible. For example, he says, don't just tell yourself you won't drink when you meet your friend at the bar. Instead, get more detailed and say: "When my friend asks if I want a drink, I'm going to say, 'No, I'm really trying not to drink for the next month to see if it changes my health,' or whatever the reason may be," he says. "Having that planned out is thought to be more effective than just having a general goal like, 'I don't want to drink.'" With a detailed strategy to keep your goal on track, you are much better equipped to handle and defeat the temptation.

3. **Practice defeating your habit in as many different contexts as you can.** Whatever we do or whichever strategy we employ to get over a habit is fragile and sensitive to small changes in the world, Russell says. The example he uses is smoking. If you learn to stop smoking in your house but then go to a bar and face your trigger, you'll be tempted to smoke. To build your habit-breaking muscle, "you want to try to do it in as many contexts as possible," he says. That's where having a detailed strategy thought through in advance will help. Knowing how sensitive your best-laid plans are to small changes in your environment should also remind you to be extra vigilant in a new context or situation where you haven't practiced overriding the habit. "Watch out for the triggers and try to short-circuit the habit before it ever gets turned on."

4. **Track and monitor how well your strategy is working.** "Whenever someone is trying to change a behavior, it's really important to monitor how well it's going," Russell

> says. It can be as simple as writing things down in a journal or on your phone or downloading an app to track your progress—and depending on your goal, there are all kinds of free and paid options out there. A few to check out: Habitica, Streaks, stickK, and Strides. "It's easy to fool yourself and remember things differently than they actually were," he says, but tracking your daily progress will help keep your monitoring glasses crystal clear. The results will work in one of two ways: give you a boost when you see your efforts have succeeded, or indicate you may need to change your approach if your strategy has not helped you reach your goal.

Chatting with Russell, I quickly realized why—and how, where, and when—I failed at cutting back my drinking when I came up with my vague intention to just "drink less." Not only was my goal wishy-washy, but I had made no attempt to remove my habit triggers or cues from my life. I kept buying alcohol and stocking our wine cabinet as I always had and making happy-hour plans with friends at restaurants or cocktail bars where I'd be faced with the substance I crave. Even if I told myself I'd cut back or abstain in those situations, something I wanted to do when we met during the work week, I didn't have a reply ready for saying no to a drink.

I wasn't tracking my intake during this period, either. It wouldn't have shown progress in the right direction anyway, a clear sign I needed to change my habit-breaking approach.

This time around and buoyed by Russell's advice, I started with a small, easy step: researching apps that would help me create a concrete goal, monitor my progress, and, ideally, break my habit but allow me to still enjoy alcohol. A smart move, according to someone specializing in helping women overcome addictive disorders. "Using an app is a great approach to reducing or stopping drinking because there's an accountability there so you don't have to rely on yourself," says Dr. Reagan Wetherill, who, among other things, is an assistant professor of psychiatry and a licensed clinical psychologist at the University of Pennsylvania Perelman School of Medicine. "They're based on cognitive behavioral therapy, which is evidence-based, and they help you set a goal but also remind you of *why* you want to reduce your drinking. They give you daily motivation, ask you to record your drinking, and then show your progress over time."

I'd reached out to Reagan after stumbling upon a study she co-authored about alcohol's effects on brain age. The *Penn Today* headline about the study—"One alcoholic drink a day linked with reduced brain size"—caught my attention, for obvious reasons. I'd known about alcohol-related health risks such as cancer and heart disease for years. But alcohol-related brain shrinkage? That was news to me. Indeed, her 2022 study found that even one alcoholic drink a day was linked with reduced brain size—and going from one to two drinks a day causes changes in the brain equivalent to aging two years. Two years! Not surprisingly, heavier drinking leads to more damage.

I don't want to dwell too much on alcohol, as this chapter is meant to help you break habits of any kind. But given how booze is so woven into today's society and present in our daily lives—not to mention a hot topic lately amongst my friends and colleagues—discussing its effects on how we age seems prudent. Especially if we want to protect our "money-makers," as Reagan refers to brains.

To be clear, even non-drinkers lose brain volume as they age, she says. It's a natural part of getting older. But as she and her colleagues found in their large-scale study involving more than 36,000 adults, alcohol accelerates the rate at which our brains shrink. Drinking, then, leads our brains to age faster than usual. Beyond causing our gray matter to shrink, our white matter is affected, too. "Alcohol messes up the tracks in the brain, the roads where information flows. It's like you're causing potholes in your roads," she says. "You'll see some of that with aging anyway, but when you consume alcohol regularly, even at moderate doses, you see more deterioration of the lovely brain you had when you were 25."

Ugh. Those findings bummed me out.

Even Reagan was bummed.

Though she's never been a big drinker, she recognizes alcohol plays a big role in how many of us socialize—and the challenges we face when we try to cut back. In the Philadelphia suburb she calls home, for example, neighbors get together for drinks, and she loves to host dinners with friends or meet them out for a bite. Alcohol is usually involved. So, the big question: Does she still drink?

Yes. Usually one to two drinks max and always with her findings in mind.

"Whenever I have a sip, I immediately think of my brain and that helps me moderate," she says. "Back when I was younger, I never thought about these things. Now I am really mindful about what I put in my body because I see the effects of alcohol every day. I can look at a brain and say, 'That person drinks.'"

Reagan's choice to drink mindfully works for her. What works for you may be different. As she says, people respond to different things and set different goals for themselves: "I think it depends on where you are in your life and what you want." Russell agrees. Unless a habit drives you to do things you don't want to do or harms you psychologically, physically, or in any way, your habit may not need breaking or taming. As he says, "If your habit of drinking two glasses of wine a night isn't causing you distress or any health problems*, then it's not clear that it's a bad habit."

(*Um, sorry to have put a damper on that illusion.)

Your needs and goals will differ from mine, your friends', your colleagues'. But if you want to scale back on your drinking—or curb any vice causing you distress or harm—using an app is an excellent starting point, the experts agree. One Reagan often recommends is I Am Sober, a free program designed to help you quit any activity or substance.

Another thing she suggests to anyone trying to overcome a habit but struggling with triggers: Ride the craving or substitute. "Cravings aren't forever. Give yourself five to ten seconds, breathe, and acknowledge you really want to do X, Y, or Z," says Reagan, "or find something else to do that's pleasurable." Pick up a book you enjoy, go for a walk, practice yoga. Heck, clean the bathroom if that's something you enjoy. Whether you ride the urge out or give your mind something else to focus on, you *can* overcome a craving. "Before you know it, the craving will be gone."

After chatting with our experts, I explored I Am Sober but decided it wasn't for me. My goal isn't to be sober and eliminate alcohol completely but, like Reagan, to cut back and drink mindfully. Eventually I landed on Reframe, "an alcohol reduction program built on the foundations of habit change, psychology, and neuroscience." According to its website, 91 percent of users report substantial decreases in alcohol use within three months. Though the app's yearly membership wasn't cheap—I paid $96.99—I was willing to front the cost. The program offered all the features I was looking for, so spending $100 to improve my physical and mental health seemed a small price to pay.

With Reframe on my phone, the experts' advice in mind, and, most importantly, my commitment to break the alcohol habit I'd established, I was ready to begin.

First, and after some loose math about the amount of alcohol I'd been consuming, I used Reframe to set a concrete, measurable goal: to have seven or fewer drinks per week. Seven alcoholic drinks would reduce my consumption and make me a guideline-abiding citizen if I lived in the United States. I wouldn't be meeting Canada's strict suggestion, but hey, you can't please everyone. Reframe then told me what I had to look forward to a year from starting the program: $10,400 saved, 55,692 empty calories saved, 1,825 REM sleep cycles added. Those numbers were motivating in themselves.

Next, I spent a lot of time thinking about how to set boundaries in my new relationship with alcohol. Reducing what I consumed from Monday to Thursday was the clear move. I started by removing triggers, which meant not buying as much wine to keep at home and planning coffee-and-walk dates with my friends instead of happy hours. Those changes were easy to implement, and as I repeat the behaviors more, they're my new norm.

Learning to ride the craving or substitute has also helped me reduce my consumption. Because though Cam and I agreed to quit drinking at home during the week, we still felt the craving. Instead of trying to ignore it, I learned to acknowledge my urge to drink and then decide to ride it out—I legit picture myself surfing a small wave—or substitute with an alternative drink. Turns out having a Diet Coke or Fresca satisfies my want for a tasty beverage and helps me move past the urge to have an alcoholic drink. Most recently, I've also started to explore the world of mocktails and alcohol-free wine. Though I have yet to discover one I love, I'm encouraged there are more options hitting the market. (Patiently waiting for Katy Perry's line of non-alcoholic aperitifs, De Soi, to come to Canada.)

I'm also lucky and grateful my husband wants to break the habit we developed together. I admit it's much easier to change when the person you share a home with wants to change, too. Having an accountability partner—in him, but also the app I use to record my drinks—is a major bonus. And it's certainly worth seeking out that kind of support from a friend, family member, or online community, no matter your goal. Because as Reframe mentions, "Research shows that having support from a friend or peer increases our chances of sticking to behaviors that align with our goals."

Having someone to share your wins with feels good, too. In the early days of our habit-changing experiment, realizing we could nix a cocktail or glass of wine and still have a great meal—and, likely, a better night overall—without alcohol was a welcome affirmation we could do it. We could change. And we felt motivated to keep going.

Having those types of successful experiences help people change habits, Russell says. Because aside from the real, dopamine-driven cravings we experience, we also tend to build up thoughts around certain habits, like "I need it" or "I have to have it." But every time we override the urge to indulge in a craving and realize we don't actually need it and we're okay without it, we begin to change our thoughts. Let's use happy hour as an example. "It's good practice to not do it and see how you respond," Russell says. "If you start to shake, that's a bad thing. But if you respond by saying, 'Wow, tonight's maybe not as exciting, but it's fine. I didn't fall apart.' That's a good experience to have to help modify those cognitions."

While I was making initial strides at reducing my weekday consumption, I knew myself well enough to know I'd need to make exceptions to my rule. And I decided early on to allow myself those moments and enjoy them without guilt, especially if I drink mindfully. Like on a recent Wednesday night when I had dinner with girlfriends I hadn't seen in ages. We dressed up, went to a great restaurant, and ordered a bottle of wine to share. But instead of having two glasses as I would have in the past, I had one glass, savored it, and then stuck to water.

Reframe applauds reductions, no matter the amount. "Be realistic about the boundaries you can uphold. You might not be able to cut back as far as you'd like right now, and that's okay," said one of the app's daily readings. "Start off with small changes. Instead of drinking three drinks at a party, have two." Whenever I choose to drink now, I strive to do just that. Having one or two fewer drinks than the old Michelle would have, no matter the situation, still allows me to enjoy alcohol while keeping me moving toward my goal.

The strategy takes some forethought, though.

Following Russell's advice, I plan what I'll say when offered a drink and want to say no. Depending on the situation and crowd

I'll be with, it can be as simple as, "No, thanks." No explanation needed. But if I'm with friends or people who know me well, my reply is along these lines: "Thanks, but I'm good. I'm trying to cut back on alcohol." And then I take my planning one step further. I envision a short answer for when someone asks me why: "I'm experimenting with drinking less to see how I feel." Short and to the point. I realize it's not my duty to defend or explain my choice, but this way I'm ready to respond if someone is curious. Choosing to not drink in many different environments is, as Russell suggested, also helping me build and flex my muscle to say no to drinks in all kinds of situations.

Thanks to all these changes, I do meet my goal most weeks. But I'm not perfect. Things like girls' nights out, a celebratory dinner with Cam involving cocktails and a bottle of wine, and weekends away mean I sometimes blow through my target. I don't beat myself up, because I know I'm still moving in the right direction and being more mindful of why and how much I'm drinking.

Here's how dramatic the shift has been: Two months into my habit-breaking experiment, we were in Mexico for a week-long family vacation. I gave myself permission to drink all the margaritas and drinks I wanted without guilt. But something crazy happened: I didn't want to drink like I used to. Sure, I had margaritas by the pool most days—and had one boozier day at a beach club—but I drank far less than the old me. It was wild and indicated how far my thoughts and feelings about alcohol have come.

The effects of my new mindset are apparent both within the app and in my life. Reframe shows my drinking has trended down, but the real, tangible effects I notice are the most motivating. I'm sleeping better. I have less anxiety after a night out with friends. I feel less foggy. I'm spending less money on alcohol. As for my urge to have happy hour on the regular? It's happening less and less. The craving is subsiding, fading with every passing week.

I won't lie.

I still love to drink wine—and bubbles, margaritas, and other cocktails. But the pandemic-induced routine we fell into to drink out of habit and not enjoyment has been tamed, subdued, squashed. Not only do I feel the craving less, I give much more thought to when and how much I'll drink because I want my actions to align with my goal to live healthier and feel great.

Landing on a balance that works for me and my lifestyle feels fantastic. Because although I could optimize *every* aspect of my life, like cutting out all sugar, salt, caffeine, and alcohol, my quality of life would suffer. I believe in finding balance, a happy medium, and right now mine includes seven drinks a week. But who knows? Maybe one day I'll cut out alcohol completely and join the sober curious movement I see popping up in mainstream media and on my Instagram feed. For now, I'm content to keep alcohol in my life and savor the sips I choose to enjoy.

There will be times I'll mess up, no doubt. I'll fail at my weekly goal or drink too much at a party or feel the pull to indulge more often. You will likely make some missteps, too, as you try to conquer your vice. It's okay, Russell says. The key is remembering not to be too hard on ourselves when it happens. "Hopefully, learning that habits are fundamental to how our brains work makes people feel not quite so bad about how hard it is for them to change their behavior," he says. "It shouldn't absolve you of needing to make the change, but it should make you have a little more empathy for yourself and others trying to change."

Treat yourself with compassion and grace—and keep moving toward your goal. We can do this, gals.

As for me, with one vice tamed but more to go, I'm contemplating trying to break a habit that's not doing my financial well-being any favors: online shopping.

Wish me luck.

THE CHEAT SHEET

- The easiest way to break a habit is to stop it from being triggered in the first place. Identify your triggers and try to remove them from your life, as best you can.
- Establish a detailed plan on how you'll behave when faced with your trigger, especially if it's in an environment where you haven't practiced overriding your habit. Get specific with what you'll say and do because that's more effective than having a vague intention.
- Practice defeating your habit in as many different situations as you can. Strategies to override habits are fragile and sensitive to small changes, so put them to work in as many situations as possible. When you find yourself in new places, situations, and contexts, be extra vigilant to avoid triggers.
- Ride the craving or substitute. Cravings don't last forever, so give yourself time to breathe, acknowledge the urge, and let it pass or find something else to do that's enjoyable, even for five minutes. Before you know it, the craving will be gone.
- Track your progress in breaking a bad habit or establishing a new one using any way that works for you, be it jotting down notes on your phone, writing in your journal, or using an app. Some app options to explore, no matter your habit: Habitica, Streaks, stickK, and Strides. If your goal is to curb or quit drinking, check out Reframe, a paid app, or I Am Sober, a free app designed to help you quit any activity or substance.
- Give yourself grace when you're trying to break a habit and extend the same to people trying to change their behaviors. Habits are fundamental to how our brains work, and they're hard to break. That doesn't absolve us from needing to make a change, but it is a reminder to have empathy for yourself when you embark on a habit-taming journey.

CHAPTER EIGHT

Get More Shuteye, Stat

As I get older, sleep is an ever-elusive bitch.

My kids sometimes wake me up, sure, but I can't blame them. My brain is the problem. Some nights, I can't fall asleep because I'm thinking about work or something I said to a friend or the errands I need to tackle the next day. Other nights, I fall asleep easily but wake up and cannot get back to sleep no matter what I try.

It's frustrating because sleep and I used to the best of friends. I could sleep anywhere, anytime, in any condition. On a plane, train, or automobile? Lights out. After a night of partying and drinking with friends? Snoozeville. Snuggled up with my husband in a full-size bed, which is only meant for one person, at my family's cabin? No problem.

Long gone are those precious days.

Now, I'm a finicky sleeper. Some people, like family members who have dealt with my requests when I'm in their home or they're in mine, might consider me high maintenance. (Sorry, Mom and Dad.) That's because everything must be just so, the conditions prime for a good night's sleep. I need a sound machine, cool and ultra-dark room, space to spread out in bed. Reading for at least ten minutes before bed is also key. If I'm not able to read a novel and calm my brain—or one thing is off in my environment, like if I can hear noise from another floor or the outside world or I'm feeling anxious or too warm—I struggle to fall asleep and stay that way. And since having kids, I'm such a light sleeper that even the smallest disturbances are enough to wake me up.

The difference between my old and new self is stark. To illustrate: Whereas I used to pass out and sleep well in shared hotel rooms on girls' trips, I recently booked my own room for an upcoming getaway with friends. I'll miss the girl talk and laughs that happen in a shared space, but I know that if I don't sleep solo, I won't sleep well. And then I'll be miserable.

I can't pinpoint when exactly my relationship with sleep shifted, but the experts have a pretty good hunch as to why many women in their late thirties to late forties struggle to get a good night's rest. One such expert is Dr. Jennifer Martin, a clinical psychologist who is board-certified in behavioral sleep medicine by the American Academy of Sleep Medicine, an organization for which she serves as president of the board of directors. She is also a professor of medicine at the David Geffen School of Medicine at the University of California, Los Angeles, and much of her work is focused on how sleep impacts health and well-being. Of particular interest to us, dear readers, her expertise includes treatments to help women with insomnia or anyone having a hard time catching Zs.

The first question I asked her when we spoke was: What happens to women's sleep as we age?

Sleep, she said, is one of those things at the intersection of sex and gender. There are real, biological differences between men and women in sleep, but there are different societal and social expectations around our sleep, too.

Sleep is similar for boys and girls during adolescence, a time when our internal circadian clocks shift later. In our twenties, we all generally move to a more central, socially standard bedtime and rise time, and as we age, it shifts even earlier. "Some people think of that as stereotyping older people, but there really is a biological phenomenon where older people have a tendency to fall asleep earlier and wake up earlier," she said. "It's just normal aging and development."

But the biggest changes for women in sleep happen around menopause—and a lot of it has to do with sleep apnea, a disorder in which people don't breathe well when they're sleeping. Though it's more common in men, Jennifer says sleep apnea rates triple in women after menopause. Estrogen and progesterone protect against sleep apnea in women, so as our hormone levels drop with age, our sleep apnea risk goes up. She says women in their forties typically don't experience major sleep issues due to hormone changes, as we still have enough on board to keep us protected, but many start to experience symptoms. Another biological factor that women often contend with in their forties is weight gain associated with perimenopause, and excess weight can cause sleep apnea.

Beyond the biological changes we face, there are other factors at play impacting our sleep. Jennifer says the data isn't consistent, but it often shows stress disrupts women's sleep more than men's sleep. That's not a surprise from an evolutionary perspective since women have largely been responsible throughout history for taking care of tiny humans that can't fend for themselves, even though we don't face the same stressors as in ancient times. "In terms of the survival of the human race, it would make sense that you're easily awakened so you can care for your offspring," Jennifer says. "We're wired to be awake in the face of danger."

Not only are women more prone to waking up, we still carry the bulk of the caregiving load in most family units. "Women have more family responsibilities than men. It's changing, but it's still not balanced," she says. And though she says the relationship to sleep within same-sex relationships isn't as well understood, there is usually a primary caregiver with more responsibilities to manage between the end of the workday and bedtime. And the primary caregivers, no matter the shape of a family, often have a harder time winding down for sleep and putting the day to rest.

If those factors weren't enough, consider the unique position many women are in today—and the stress that comes along with it. "Women in this age range are often caring for children *and* parents. And, at this point in their professional lives, there are critical career milestones," Jennifer says. "It's this constellation of psychosocial factors, all at the same time, and this might be the first generation where that's happening because we had kids later than our parents."

You could say we're trailblazers. Down a trail that leads to less, worse sleep.

But striving to get enough good sleep on the regular should be one of our top priorities, if not our number-one priority. The benefits of sleep are profound. Among other things, it can help us:

- Boost our immunity, so that we get sick less often.
- Protect our metabolic, mental, and cardiovascular health.
- Stay at a healthy weight.
- Think clearly, perform well at work, and better manage stress.
- Recover from workouts, repairing our muscles and recharging our bodies.
- Feel well rested and refreshed.

The importance of sleep to our overall health and well-being can't be overstated even when stacked up against other pillars such as nutrition, fitness or body movement, and stress management. Here's what Dr. Krista Scott-Dixon, the former director of curriculum at Precision Nutrition and the co-author of Girls Gone Strong's new Menopause Coaching Specialist Certification, had to say about sleep: "Sleep is the rock star. It's the master metabolic regulator. It controls and manages all the aspects of your metabolism, so if you're not sleeping well or enough, your nutrition is screwed, your appetite and hunger are screwed, your digestion is screwed, your insulin sensitivity is screwed, you're screwed."

That's a whole bunch of screwed. And it doesn't end there.

"Without good sleep, your ability to execute movement is impaired, you don't recover, and your muscles don't get that growth and repair. And your ability to manage your mindset is significantly inhibited, which has other implications for things like being in a relationship with a partner, parenting, being effective at work, all that stuff," Krista says. "So, if we're thinking about the pie chart of where you should be placing your attention, it should be much more on sleep than anything else."

Sleep really is a rock star.

Let's figure out how to optimize it and maybe sneak more into our schedules, especially if "refreshed and well rested" aren't words in your vocabulary.

To start, it might help to set some realistic expectations. Hint: Perfection is not the goal.

"We aim for five nights a week where you're content with your sleep, not seven. It's not going to be perfect every night," says Dr. Shelby Harris, a licensed clinical psychologist specializing in behavioral sleep medicine and a specialist in cognitive behavioral therapy who wrote *The Women's Guide to Overcoming Insomnia: Get a Good Night's Sleep Without Relying on Medication*. Shelby says even she has a bad night's sleep every now and then, and that's totally normal.

To her, quality over quantity of sleep is the most important thing to tackle first because, as we all know, it's sometimes hard to find more time for sleep. Not only that, giving people a set target of hours to hit every night adds pressure, which is the last thing we need.

Jennifer agrees. She says she hesitates to share a target for the number of hours of sleep women should get a night, especially if they struggle with insomnia, because then hitting that number almost becomes something they must work at. "When, really, what you have to do is go to bed and just let sleep happen to you," she says. We shouldn't get *too* fixated on how many hours we're getting. Rather, we should focus on how we feel throughout the day, she says. "But I think people are tempted to go buy some kind of a tracker, wear it and measure their sleep, and then freak out if they're not getting seven hours."

Why seven?

Because seven hours a night seems to be the magic number. Jennifer and Shelby say the recommended range is seven to nine hours a night, but they emphasize that it's *just* a range. Everyone will have different sleep needs for feeling well rested and refreshed. But if we want to reap the many health benefits of sleep, it's clear: We need to get seven or more hours of shuteye a night. As Jennifer sums it up, "Most people need seven or more to feel well and to be well."

With this general guideline in mind—and the awareness that it's not realistic for anyone to sleep perfectly or get enough sleep every single night—let's chat about some healthy sleep habits that can set you up for success, otherwise known as sleep hygiene. Here are some habits the Centers for Disease Control and Prevention recommend for improving your sleep health:

- Be consistent. Go to bed at the same time each night and get up at the same time each morning, including on the weekends.
- Make sure your bedroom is quiet, dark, relaxing, and at a comfortable temperature.
- Remove electronic devices, such as TVs, computers, and smartphones, from the bedroom.
- Avoid large meals, caffeine, and alcohol before bedtime.
- Get some exercise. Being physically active during the day can help you fall asleep more easily at night.

By now, most of us have heard those tips ad nauseam—in women's magazines, on podcasts, from parents who cut out articles and leave them in your old bedroom for the next time you come to visit (thanks, Mom and Dad). Doesn't mean we're good at following that advice to a T, though.

As for me, I've excelled on the bedroom front, creating an ideal sleeping oasis over the last few years. Our master bedroom is cool, ultra dark at night thanks to the blackout shades we installed a few years ago, and free of electronic devices (yes, even our phones). But I'm not always great at avoiding screens before bed—or alcohol, for that matter, on nights out with friends. On those occasions when I drink too close to bedtime, I pay the price with disrupted, hot, anxious sleep. Whatever. Even our experts have confirmed perfection isn't realistic.

We can always improve our sleep habits—and thanks to the following seven tips from Jennifer and Shelby that go beyond basic sleep hygiene, we have the strategies we need to execute. Here are their suggestions on how to optimize the quality and amount of your sleep:

1. **Choose to make sleep a priority, whether you live alone, with a partner, or with your family.** Create a culture around sleep, says Jennifer, and make decisions that enable a consistent, early enough bedtime to meet your needs and those of your loved ones. When her kids were young, for example, she implemented a household rule: No television on school nights. Not only did this free up time for shared, meaningful activities, it helped everyone go to bed earlier. Though her kids are older now and she has no control over their TV habits, they have retained the awareness and mindset that sleep is important. "They both know they feel better when they get enough sleep," she says. Whether you live on your own or with others, choosing to make sleep a priority and something you *actually do* is paramount for your well-being and theirs.

2. **Keep a consistent bedtime and wake time, with ninety minutes fluctuation max.** Gone are the days of our twenties, when we'd often stay out late, no matter the night, and sleep in for hours on the weekend. As we get older, our bodies crave routine and structure—and our circadian rhythm needs that routine, too, Shelby says. "Keeping a more consistent bedtime and wake time with ninety minutes max fluctuation is, in my opinion, the biggest gold standard. If you can do that, you'll help keep a lot of other problems at bay." But again, don't worry if you're not perfect on this front. Shelby says, "Just try to be as consistent as you can."

3. **Think of your day as having seventeen hours, not twenty-four, and plan accordingly.** One of the strategies Jennifer often recommends to clients is to stop thinking about a day as having twenty-four hours. "Take seven hours out for sleep, think of your day as having seventeen hours, and plan those hours. I use seven because that's the minimum that most people need," she says, adding that she needs closer to eight to feel well rested, efficient, and smart. Removing those sleep hours from your day, be it seven, eight, or nine, and adjusting your schedule to accommodate those non-negotiable hours will help you prioritize sleep and make the most of your waking hours. "Once you're getting a good amount of sleep, it's amazing how much more you can get done in the time you have."

4. **Spend five minutes every day on a mindfulness meditation of your choice.** Whether you focus on your breathing, imagine yourself in a peaceful setting like a meadow or beach, or even stare out the window to observe and describe what you see, meditating for just five minutes a day will help you calm your brain at night and wind down for a good night's rest. But don't wait until bedtime

to give this a try. "People often think we mean listen to a sleepcast or meditation to fall asleep, but that's not it. It's about spending five minutes earlier in your day practicing any kind of meditation," Shelby says. "When people just do it at night before bed, it's harder if you haven't practiced during the day. There's more at stake, in a weird way, because you're trying to force yourself to sleep." And the more you meditate, the stronger your mental muscle will become. "You'll get better at noticing when your brain is busy and letting it go," she says. "Then at night, you can let go easier because you've put the work in at the gym, essentially, during the day."

5. **Incorporate twenty minutes of "worry time" into your evening routine.** If you're anxious and have endless worries, give "worry time" a try. Here's what Shelby recommends you do every evening, but not right before bed: Sit down with a pen and paper, set a timer for twenty minutes, and write down every worry that's on your mind. "It's like a brain dump," she says, adding you can use that time to just write down your worries and even take care of some of them if you want to. Either way, when the timer goes and your twenty minutes are up, worry time is over. That means when a worry pops up at any other time of day—be it morning, bedtime, or in the middle of the night—tell yourself, "Not now, during worry time." Doing this help will help keep your worries from running rampant all day and quiet your mind when it's time to sleep. Shelby says, "Essentially, you're training yourself to sit and worry, almost needlessly, during that time as opposed to at any other time."

6. **Make your bedroom a pleasing space to be.** Walk in your bedroom and think about how you feel there, Jennifer says. Do you feel calm? Relaxed? Is the space inviting? Your

room is where you go to sleep, so it should feel pleasant to be there, she says. Things like keeping your room tidy, making your bed every morning, and avoiding clutter will help. (For tips on how to declutter, see Megan Golightly's tips in chapter 10.) Jennifer says, "You don't have to necessarily redecorate the whole room, but it's amazing what a fresh coat of paint and some new bedding can do."

7. **Do not, ever, under any circumstances, have a TV in your bedroom.** You've heard it before (and above!), but have you listened to the advice? Because the experts strongly, *strongly* recommend you nix having a TV in your bedroom. "It's my no-exceptions rule," Jennifer says. "I have never once heard of a TV in a master bedroom or a kid's bedroom helping people sleep better." Same goes for phones, although Jennifer has given up on telling people to get their phones out of their rooms. If you must keep your phone close by, she suggests turning off all your alerts and keeping it out of arm's reach. Shelby hasn't given up the phone fight yet, and recommends families create a charging section somewhere in the house that forces everyone to charge their phones outside their bedrooms. And don't try pulling the "I use my phone as my alarm clock" excuse with Shelby. "Get an old-school alarm clock. You don't need anything fancy," she says. "I use the same alarm clock I've had since high school."

I, for one, hated my high school alarm clock. It did the trick, yes, but I detested its harsh, beeping sound. If you do too, then I have a suggestion. It's an alarm clock that veers on the fancy side, but it's been worth every penny. For years, and based on the recommendation from a sleep expert I once interviewed about sleep hygiene, I have used the Philips Wake-up Light, a sunrise-simulating light that gradually increases in intensity and color, going from a soft red to warm orange to bright yellow. You can have nature sounds or the radio kick in at a certain time, but the light usually wakes me well before any sound comes on.

Ladies, I love this contraption so much. Waking up to a soft, glowing light instead of an urgent, repetitive beep is divine, and much kinder to my pre-coffee brain. Check it out if that kind of wakeup appeals to you, too. And I should note, I do set my alarm for the same time every day of the work week, with a thirty-minute fluctuation max, and I have a consistent bedtime, too. I've been *so* consistent for so long that I wake at the same time—without an alarm—even when I don't have to. It's kind of annoying. But the next time I find myself awake at 6 a.m. while on vacation, I'll remind myself I've achieved Shelby's gold standard. And then seek coffee.

Though I'm waking the same way as always, I've made a few changes to my daily routine and sleep setup since speaking with Jennifer and Shelby. First, I invested in new sheets and a cloud-like comforter (the Organic Cotton Puff Comforter from Parachute, to be precise), making our bed extra inviting and cozy. I love being in our bed—and that's a feeling worth striving for, says Jennifer, because not only is it wonderful to physically enjoy our surroundings, but we want our brains to know our bedrooms are for true rest and relaxation.

On that note, let's quickly address the twenty-minute sleep rule you've probably heard by now: If you can't fall asleep after twenty minutes, you should get out of bed, move to a couch or someplace cozy to read or do something that's not too stimulating, and then head back to bed when you feel ready to try again. It's a decent rule to keep in mind, says Jennifer, but she has a caveat: "If you're in bed, cozy and happy, and you're awake, but you don't care, just stay there. You don't need to be too excited about getting out of bed after twenty minutes," she says. "But once you're struggling and upset, that's the time to grab a blanket and go sit on the couch. We don't want you to walk into your room and have the subconscious association that this is where you struggle."

Whereas I used to have a hard time shutting my brain down in the middle of the night, sometimes spiraling into anxious thoughts and then getting out of bed because I was so frustrated, I'm getting better at calming my brain and falling back asleep faster. I credit my daily mindfulness practice—and that's the second big change I made.

Though I'd already incorporated meditation into my daily routine (see chapter 9 for more details), after speaking with Shelby and Jennifer I started setting my alarm for fifteen minutes earlier than usual to prioritize meditating for five to ten minutes. Insight Timer, the free app I use to guide my mindfulness practice, has a whole section dedicated to short, effective morning meditations. Making time to meditate before the craziness of everyday life kicks in is helping me stick to a daily practice. Also, I'm starting my day on a serene note, especially when the meditation is one that helps me feel centered, focused, and joyful.

Practicing quieting my thoughts every morning is helping me do the same at night. The more I meditate, the easier it's becoming to shut down anxious thoughts before they take hold and keep me awake. I also feel calmer at bedtime, like I'm not as "wired for danger." Overall, I'm having an easier time letting sleep wash over me, just happen with ease—a thrilling development after spending years feeling like I had to hunt sleep down.

Third, my husband and I decided to implement a no-TV rule on Tuesday and Wednesday nights. It's not as hardcore as Jennifer's but a step in the right direction. What's wild is I grew up with the same rule—no TV at all from Monday to Thursday—and my brother and I were *not* fans at the time. Now, I'm grateful to my parents for making that unpopular decision and prioritizing our health and well-being. When I drew inspiration from them and Jennifer, suggesting to my husband, Cam, that we nix our kids' TV time altogether on weeknights, he was skeptical we could pull it off. Frankly, I was too. Mostly because we consider our kids' TV time much needed "us time."

Despite our best efforts over the years, our kids go to bed late by kid standards, falling asleep close to 9 p.m. We like to be in bed shortly after. That means our window for quality family time every night is big, but our window to do anything sans kiddos is small. Giving them thirty minutes of TV time means we can sit, read, zone out on social media, or have a dip in the hot tub together. Some nights, we use that time to tackle household chores. Either way, our kids' TV time has felt as necessary for us as much as them.

Based on the results from our experiment, though, we're feeling encouraged to make some changes.

When we first cut out TV on Tuesday and Wednesday nights, there was some grumbling, moaning, and general malaise amongst the child folk. However, they moved on quickly, realizing they had more time to play mini sticks (with Cam), shoot hoops in the backyard (with me), or mix weird potions using every toothpaste, shampoo, conditioner, hair gel, and soap they could find in our bathrooms (together, while whispering). Cam and I also realized that (duh) we could just focus on ourselves for a bit *while the kids were still awake,* and they would find ways to entertain themselves (see: weird potions).

Most importantly, something remarkable happened: On those TV-free nights, our munchkins were ready for bed and asleep thirty minutes earlier than usual, a natural shift we didn't even push for. We went to bed earlier those nights, too, yet still had more time to ourselves before lights out. So yes, the experiment has gone well, and we will be keeping our two weeknights TV-free.

Now, you may be wondering, and rightly so, given the positive results, are we considering nixing TV *every* weeknight? Hell no. At least not anytime soon. My end-of-the-day, weary soul still looks forward to the reprieve TV time affords us as parents, however brief and ill advised. Furthermore, what are we? Some kind of parental heroes? We need screens now and then!

Something I don't need, I've discovered, is worry time. The first evening I sat down to "brain dump" all my worries onto paper, I exhausted my list after four minutes. The next night, one minute. Turns out I don't have hundreds of worries so much as a busy mind. And that could be a helpful distinction if you're unsure what you need most. "Meditation is great for anybody because you don't have to be anxious or worried to benefit. If your brain is just busy and you're thinking about the day at bedtime, that's when meditation is really helpful," Shelby says. "But for people who have endless worries, worry time is a really good thing for them to do."

Another thing we should do is differentiate between the occasional bad night of sleep and insomnia, a common sleep disorder. If you're having a hard time falling asleep or staying asleep, how often does it happen and how long has it been going on? Insomnia, says Jennifer, is when you struggle to sleep more than three times a week, it's been happening for more than three months, and it's impacting how you feel and function during the day.

How you're feeling during your waking hours is key because some people can get by on less sleep than others, say the experts. If you routinely get six hours of sleep and feel great, then you likely don't have a disorder. But if you're tossing and turning at night, feeling foggy during the day, showing other physical symptoms, and stressed about your lack of sleep, you could have insomnia or another underlying sleep disorder. If the latter situation sounds like you (hang in there, girl), here are a few tips to keep in mind:

1. **Avoid the quick fix.** If you're struggling with sleep and can't get back on track on your own, resist the urge to look for a quick fix, advises Jennifer. "The temptation is to go buy some over-the-counter melatonin at a drugstore," she says. "And melatonin is used for some very specific sleep disorders, but it doesn't work any better than a placebo for insomnia." In short, quick fixes won't solve the underlying issue. But the suggestion in tip #2 might.
2. **Download and try Insomnia Coach, a free app for anyone suffering from insomnia.** Jennifer recommends

Insomnia Coach, an app based on cognitive behavioral therapy, to anyone struggling with insomnia (including her friends). She estimates a quarter of people with insomnia can get their sleep back on track using the app, which includes a guided training plan to help track and improve sleep, personal feedback about your sleep, fun sleep tips, an interactive sleep diary, and more. "Try the app," she recommends, "and if it doesn't work, go see somebody."

3. **Talk to a sleep specialist.** When hearing about women's sleep troubles, many primary care doctors are still inclined to simply give handouts on sleep hygiene, prescribe a sleeping pill, suggest giving melatonin a try, or even dismiss sleep issues as anxiety or depression. The truth is, says Shelby, you could have insomnia, mild sleep apnea, restless leg syndrome, a hormonal issue, or something else keeping you awake. "It could be a million different things" Shelby says. "You are the expert on you. If you feel like something is off, find someone who will fully evaluate you." As for where, you have options. The experts recommend finding a sleep center (at sleepeducation.org), a psychologist who's certified in behavioral sleep medicine (at behavioralsleep.org), or a specialist in menopause care (at menopause.org). Whatever you choose, don't wait too long if you're struggling. As Jennifer says, "The sooner you can get help, the better."

For my part, I feel grateful my sleep is back on track. My mind is easier to calm at night, and that's made all the difference. Knowing the odd night of bad sleep is normal is also relieving the pressure I used to put on myself to get a perfect sleep every night. Finally, I'm not apologizing anymore for choosing sleep, setting boundaries around my eight hours, and optimizing my sleep environment. Sleep is just too important to my health and everyday well-being to not prioritize. I guess you could say that when it comes to Krista's advice, I've got my pie-orities straight. (Oof. Sorry.)

And if, after all this, you're still not convinced that sleep is worth focusing on and making changes for, one last piece of advice from Jennifer: Write down the three most important things in your life. Now write down how your poor sleep is affecting those things. "It's a lot easier to make changes if you say, 'I want to sleep better because I want to be a better partner' or 'I want to sleep better because I value my work life and I'm not showing up how I should,'" she says. "People are not motivated by their blood pressure. They're motivated by the things they really care about."

Sleep helps us become the best version of ourselves, benefiting not just us but everything and everyone we value. That's why I hope you, too, start having an easier time falling asleep, staying that way, and, should you wake up, getting back to dreamland quickly.

Night, night, dear readers.

THE CHEAT SHEET

- Choose to make sleep a priority in your home. Setting that intention will help you keep healthy boundaries around sleep and encourage others to get the rest they need, too.
- Aim for a good night's sleep five nights out of seven—the kind of sleep that leaves you feeling refreshed, well rested, and ready for your day. Remember, the odd bad night of sleep is normal, and no one sleeps perfectly all the time.
- To reap sleep's many health benefits, aim for seven or more hours of sleep a night. Though everyone's needs will vary slightly, most adults need seven or more hours to feel well and to be well.
- Think of your day as having seventeen hours, not twenty-four. When you subtract the minimum seven hours of sleep you should be getting every night, you're left with seventeen awake, functioning hours. Plan your schedule accordingly.

- Make your bedroom a pleasing, calm space. Keep it dark, cool, and tidy. Invest in cozy bedding. And do not, under any circumstances, keep a TV in your room. No exceptions!
- Spend five minutes daily on a mindfulness meditation of your choice, ideally earlier in the day. If you wait until bedtime to meditate, you'll feel pressure to calm your brain and fall asleep.
- If you're a worrier, incorporate twenty minutes of "worry time" into your evening routine. Use that time to write down every worry on your mind and act on some if you want to. When worries pop up outside of that time, be it day or night, tell yourself, "Not now, during worry time."
- If you're struggling to sleep, download the expert-recommended Insomnia Coach app. It's like getting a sleep coach for free and will help with everything from tracking your sleep and setting new goals to quieting your mind and curbing habits that disrupt your sleep.
- You are the expert on you, and you know when something is wrong. If you've tried to get your sleep on track but can't, don't wait too long to seek help. Talk to your doctor and don't hesitate to seek out a sleep specialist.

CHAPTER NINE

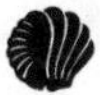

Take Your Libido and Sex Life to the Next Level

In retrospect, it's easy to define my sexual journey in eras.

My teens were when my body came alive, a thrilling season of firsts. I had my first kiss at a junior high dance. First make-out in the back of a car in high school. First time having sex, just after graduation. A year later, the first terrifying call home to tell my parents I'd be spending the night at my boyfriend's house. Bless my dad, who calmly said, "We don't support that."

I respected his answer.

I still spent the night.

My late teens were lovely as I began to understand and respect my body as a sexual being.

If my teens were for firsts, then my twenties were for seconds. I dated plenty, rotating between longer-term relationships, bouts of singledom, and shorter flings that fizzled out. While exploring the pleasure buffet, I discovered how much I loved simple, low-key indulgences. For instance, kissing was my favorite, like my ideal situation. Would the guys have agreed? Who cares! I loved it. Kissing was low on stress and commitment but high on pleasure and fun. I earned the nickname a friend gave me, The Kissing Bandit, honestly.

But exploring sexual pleasure was something I was trying on my own, too. A friend told me she was obsessed with a mini vibrator from Lelo, a company that makes luxe sex toys. I bought one, used it, and loved it for years until I accidentally threw it into the washing machine and destroyed it. Devastating. Other toys eventually came and went, but—hot tip—nothing has been as good as my Lelo clitoral massager. That is, until a recent discovery.

But more on that later.

My thirties started out with much of the same—dating, singleness, repeat—but my life took a turn when I met my husband, Cam. We flirted, he asked me out, and we had an hours-long kissing session in my car on our first date.

We eventually started having the most playful, satisfying sex of my life. That sex kept up well after we got married, a blissful time when our clothing flew off the minute we walked through the door. My lingerie budget skyrocketed. Desire coursed through me all day long.

And then we had two kids.

Suffice it to say having babies a mere twenty-two months apart didn't make me feel sexy or filled with lust. And it didn't make finding time to have sex easier. But my desire kept a pulse, and we carved out time for sex as best we could. Now our kids are seven and five years old. Life has settled into a comfortable, albeit no less demanding, groove.

I am older now, too, and as I approach my mid-forties, I feel a new sexual era is afoot. Much of it is fantastic. I know my body better than in my twenties or thirties, so I know what I like in bed. I'm more confident asking for it, too. And I'm thrilled to be married to someone I'm deeply attracted to and who is attracted to me.

Of course, there are some not-so-fantastic aspects.

My body is changing with age, an evolution I am striving to embrace and accept. I still have my issues. From seeing wrinkles appear and having persistent lower-back pain to watching my breasts sag and overcoming mild uterine prolapse following the birth of my second baby (too much information?), my body is different than before. But that's not my biggest challenge, not by a long shot. My main hurdle is finding the time and energy for sex. I mean, most days I don't even have time to *think* about sex.

Neither do many women I know. Here are a few of the things I've heard lately from the gals in my life about their sex lives:

- "My brain is always going. I'm thinking about everything I have to get done, like make lunches and fold laundry."
- "I wouldn't care if I never had sex again."
- And the most common: "Sex just feels like another thing on my to-do list."

You get the gist.

And I know you understand. Because no matter your marital status or child situation, if you're an adult woman navigating the highs and lows, the demands and stresses of everyday life, then I imagine you can relate to feeling overloaded and under-rested. These are not prime conditions for unleashing the sexual goddess within. These are conditions requiring sweatpants and early bedtimes.

A dear girlfriend recently sent me an Instagram post by @mytherapistsays that says it all:

Me at 18: As long as I get home at 4 a.m., I can get up for work at 6.

Me now: How dare you even suggest we start a movie at 8 p.m.

Our sleep needs, bodies, and daily routines have undoubtedly changed, but must our sex lives dwindle as a result? I hope not. Because, well, I enjoy sex.

But I'm also realistic. At this stage of life, I'm not aiming for sex on the daily—and if you are, then, woman, I salute you—but I would certainly feel sad if I never had it again. That's why I am deeply curious about how we, as women approaching midlife, can boost desire, experience more pleasure, and make the most of our sex lives.

We can start, says one expert, with shedding unrealistic expectations. Just like it's not realistic for many of us to stay up late anymore (goodbye, 8 p.m. movies), it's likely not realistic to have the bodies we did or the sex we had in our twenties. Accepting that is not bleak. It's freeing and can set the stage for something more.

"This is the perfect time for a renewal, a new creation of yourself as a sexual being," says Karen B.K. Chan, an award-winning Toronto-based sex and emotional literacy educator. Much of her work is dedicated to helping people overcome awkward, hard, or embarrassing feelings about sex to access greater pleasure.

She says though women often face common challenges at this stage—whether they're stuck in a sexual rut in their long-term relationships, unable to orgasm during sex, or burdened with the daily grind, among others—there are also benefits that come with greater age and self-awareness. "There's that joke that after 40 we're those people walking around naked in the change-room because we just don't care anymore. Before, there was this hyper-vigilance and super-self-consciousness. For many people, that dips at this stage of life—and that's a huge opportunity."

Learning to access pleasure can help us seize it.

Before diving into sexual pleasure, though, Karen likes to remind people that we can engage in *all kinds* of pleasures that feel good, be they rolling around naked in your sheets, having a bubble bath, scuba diving, or getting a massage. Masturbation and sex may be pleasures you enjoy. They may not be. The point is they're personal, and all that matters is that you pursue whatever brings *you* pleasure and joy. "Someone has written this narrative for us that sex is the best thing ever. For some of us, it really isn't," says Karen. "I hope that instead of feeling a big loss, you tune into what is the best shit ever. Because I hope you have more of that."

And if sex is something you have enjoyed in the past but don't crave now, then Karen has a few questions for you to consider: How was sex the last ten times you had it? Did it blow your mind? Did you feel like a new person after? If your answers are "Not awesome," "No," and "Uh, is that possible?" then don't write off pursuing sexual pleasure. All you're dealing with is a solid case of cause and effect—not a death knell for your sex life. As Karen says, "Sometimes there is low desire because what we've had is not that good."

We deserve good sex, ladies. So, for anyone who's interested in accessing more pleasure and cultivating desire, Karen has a range of things we can try. She calls it "pleasure work" and it includes:

1. **Tuning into how we feel and allowing ourselves to feel it, no matter the emotion.** Many women live with worry, anxiety, and an array of emotions we'd rather not face. To live with these emotions and function in our day-to-day lives, we do many different things, says Karen, from numbing our feelings and distracting ourselves from their presence to locking away uncomfortable thoughts to avoid them altogether. But suppressing and numbing a part of ourselves so we don't feel anything makes it hard to magically free up the part that wants to feel and experience pleasure. "If we stop to feel what's going on, and you don't even have to have words for what's going on, but just feel," says Karen, "that is pleasure work, even if none of what you feel is pleasurable."
2. **Inhabiting our bodies and owning our viewpoints during sex.** The world teaches girls to experience their sexual selves through the outside, says Karen. We are not encouraged to explore what *we* like or want. Instead, we learn to

worry if others view us as sexy and palatable. "The school of femininity teaches us to install a camera outside of ourselves, and we end up viewing ourselves that way," she says. "Many women I talk to about sex don't have internal images of them looking up at their partners. They are seeing what they think their partners are seeing." Anytime we think about sucking in our stomachs, whether our breasts look good from that angle, or how we look as we approach orgasm, we sacrifice our ability to feel pleasure. That's why learning to be more present in our bodies is such a profound opportunity. (Tips on how to do this to come!)

3. **Understanding that, for women, pleasure leads to desire—not the other way around.** Most men feel desire and then seek pleasure. But that's not necessarily how our bodies work. "For many people with clitorises, pleasure comes first," says Karen, "and then as pleasure is experienced, desire comes. This is not a narrative that gets told a lot." To experiment with the pleasure-desire sequence, Karen suggests women chat openly with partners about wanting to share small pleasures together first—things like hugging, kissing, and dancing. If desire takes over, things can progress from there. If it doesn't, we should be free to stop without feeling pressure or worrying we're letting our partners down.

My conversation with Karen gave me much to ponder. In the following weeks, I paid close attention to what I was seeing and feeling during sex and tried to dismiss any thoughts about how my body looked. I listened to my emotions and their effect on my body, one day even crawling back into bed mid-morning when I felt sad. And I told Cam I'd love more kissing, my favorite small pleasure. Sometimes things progressed, sometimes not. I enjoyed every kiss.

But where I've really excelled at following her advice is embracing the idea that sex can and should be different than in my twenties or thirties. Still satisfying and healthy, but different. To illustrate *how* different, I offer you this example: Whereas Cam and I used to have energetic, sometimes multiple-times-a-day sex, we now rely on a little something we call The Lazy Fuck.

Now, if the name doesn't give it away, this is no-frills sex. There's no prep work needed. No lit candles. No fancy moves.

This is come-as-you-are sex.

And that's what we love most about The Lazy Fuck. Because little effort is involved, it's easy to squeeze in at the end of a long day or during a busy week.

Let me tell you how this usually plays out. It's 9:45 p.m. on a Wednesday and we haven't had sex since Sunday. But we're tired. But we want to get naked. But we're so tired. When the "Friends" rerun we've just watched ends, one of us will turn to the other, raise our eyebrows, and, with a twinkle of hope in our eyes, ask, "Lazy Fuck?"

Nine times out of ten, the answer is yes because there's so little pressure. I don't need to worry about shaving my legs or putting on lingerie. Cam doesn't have to worry about . . . oh, that's right, guys don't worry about anything before sex. Regardless, we know what we're signing up for: a good but easy time.

Turns out there's a term for this type of fornication. It's classier. It's legit. And it's actually a great thing for your relationship. My friends, meet maintenance sex.

That's how psychologist Dr. Lori Brotto describes the quick, regular sex that couples in long-term relationships often end up having. You know the kind. Like when you have ten minutes to spare at bedtime or your kids are watching a television show in the other room. Those are prime opportunities to engage in maintenance sex—and squeezing it in is a good thing, says Lori. "But every once in a while, you need the special, full-meal treatment, which does require more time. That's when you can do novel things, bring in a toy, experiment a bit, and not worry that your kids are going to walk through the door," she says.

As Karen said, too, being present and tuning into your body is critical because, without that mental focus, it's hard to feel pleasurable sensations. And feeling pleasure is what makes sex so gratifying. But Lori told me that many women struggle to let go of their worries, to-do lists, and anxieties when they're having sex.

I'm not surprised because I'm one of them.

I sometimes find it hard to turn my brain off, especially when we have a small time window and shifting from work or mom mode isn't easy. How are we supposed to do it? How do we turn off our brains and turn on our vaginas?

Lori has suggestions.

She is not only a professor in the Department of Obstetrics and Gynecology at the University of British Columbia and the executive director of the Women's Health Research Institute; she is also a member of the International Academy of Sex Research and the Society for Sex Therapy and Research, among other organizations. She's also the author of *Better Sex Through Mindfulness: How Women Can Cultivate Desire* and *The Better Sex Through Mindfulness Workbook*. Lori is well known for her ability to help women rev their libidos and improve their sex lives.

Here is what she says typically stops women from revving at full throttle in midlife (I'm sure you're aware, but here we go):

- Hormonal changes contributing to vaginal dryness that, on its own, doesn't directly affect libido and interest in sex. But if dryness causes pain, discomfort, or loss of pleasure, that can definitely impact desire.
- A slew of relational, societal, cultural, and interpersonal changes happening as we age. And let's not forget about body-image issues as we develop wrinkles, put on weight because of estrogen fluctuations with perimenopause, or

develop new aches and pains. "We're immersed in a landscape of unrealistic beauty ideals," says Lori, "and aging is not kind to the body when we compare ourselves to those." Unfortunately, when women feel shame or embarrassment about their bodies, they often don't want their partners to touch them anymore.

- Big life events, like kids leaving home or parents passing away, can often trigger depression, anxiety, and a loss of personal identity.
- The demands of daily life—everything from performing well at work and maintaining friendships to raising kids and caring for elderly parents—are unrelenting and ever-present. They can also be exhausting. "The same gas tank you're using to fuel your daily activities is the same gas tank that fuels sexual energy," she says. "It's not a separate one."

No wonder maintenance sex is a thing.

Before we get into how to mitigate these challenges and achieve maximum pleasure on our own, with a partner, or with many partners (get it, girl), let's chat quickly about *why* sex is important. Sure, orgasms are thrilling and all, but research shows that sexually satisfied couples are more likely to report higher physical health. You may be wondering: Does better physical health lead to better sexual satisfaction or does better sexual satisfaction lead people to the gym? "We don't know," says Lori, "but do those two go together? Definitely."

Researchers also know that, for men, sexual activity can be important for maintaining prostate health and decreasing their risk for prostate cancer. For women, there is tons of evidence linking sexual satisfaction to improved mood and ability to manage stress—two things critical to overall health and well-being. So beyond having a good time while getting our rocks off, striving for sexual satisfaction is a worthy endeavor.

Let's pause to take in Lori's choice words: sexual satisfaction. Not sexual frequency.

"I say that very deliberately because you might be sexually satisfied with two great encounters a year," she says. "We need not get hung up on that number."

That makes sense. Everyone has different needs. But, if you're still a *teensy* bit curious about how much sex everyone else has, know this: Research suggests couples in long-term relationships have sex, on average, once every seven to ten days. Interestingly, people today have less sex than twenty years ago, when couples in long-term relationships had sex seven times more per year on average. Lori speculates higher levels of stress and lower levels of desire are at the heart of the decline.

Despite feeling crunched for time, Cam and I are more sexually active than the average couple—okay, on our good weeks. And though I'd deem the majority of our intimate weekday encounters as maintenance sex, we carve out time for the special, full-meal treatment every so often. We put effort in to stay connected, but there's always room for improvement. As in, I still need strategies to turn my brain *off* and my body *on.* And I'm always interested in learning tips that will enhance the sexual experience for both of us.

Speaking with Lori gave me an abundance of strategies. And after months of putting them into action, I am happy—nay, delighted!—to report they work. Oh, how they work. The best news? They don't take months to take effect. The very first time we tried one of Lori's suggestions, a mere two days after I spoke with her, Cam and I had an especially satisfying session. I interrupted our contented silence afterward to ask him what he thought. He paused for a second and then said, "I'll tell you this much: It felt *good.*"

Everyone wins with these strategies.

So, let's get to them! Here are four of Lori's top tips:

1. **Practice staying present in your body.** Lori's tool of choice is mindfulness, but she says any strategy that helps you

pay attention in the present moment will help. That could mean you follow a structured mindfulness program for ten minutes a day, learn to dismiss distracting thoughts through meditation, or spend thirty seconds every day thinking about how to be present during your next sexual encounter. The goal is to learn how to quiet the mind and enhance your mind-body connection, which can be tricky. "The kind of multitasking that allows you to get everything done in the rest of your life, unfortunately, continues during sexual activity," Lori says. Anyone whose mind has wandered during sex knows exactly what she's talking about. "You might be showing up and responding to touch, but the mind is absolutely critical for ongoing feelings of arousal and perceiving those sensations." That's why training your brain to stay more present at any time of day will, in turn, benefit your sex life.

2. **Plan sex with your partner.** Talking to a partner about sex is sometimes difficult for women, Lori says. But it's critical. So critical, in fact, that research shows sexual communication between partners is the biggest predictor of long-term sexual satisfaction. Not orgasm frequency. Not intensity of arousal. It's as simple as: Are you communicating with your partner about sex? Lori suggests starting with a conversation to plan sex for the coming days, weeks, and months and to discuss contingency plans if a scheduled session must be nixed. (Because, life.) "Try to make it a joint effort, so one person isn't always responsible," she says. "Or have one person be responsible for one month and the other the next. There should be a shared commitment to planning."

3. **Use the time in between sexual encounters to cultivate desire.** When she's working with clients, Lori often shares this dynamite insight: foreplay starts when your last sexual encounter ends. Whether that window is days, weeks,

months, or years long, one thing is for sure: We should use that time to prime ourselves for our next sexual encounter. Using a vibrator to self-stimulate, reading fantasy or erotica, listening to sexy stories, even just thinking about sex every now and then—these are all useful activities that will help ignite your body, Lori says. But to make the most of them, you must tune into your body. These activities "don't necessarily turn you on in your mind, so this is where mindfulness comes back in," she says. "If you're using one of those tools, make sure you're paying attention to your body at the same time."

4. **Always use a lubricant.** No matter what you're engaging in—touch, oral sex, penetration, masturbation with a toy, or anything else—use a lubricant. The liquid or gel commonly known as "lube" is designed to minimize friction and increase wetness. Using it just makes everything feel better, says Lori, and when you feel pleasurable sensations, desire increases. So don't let any preconceived notion about lube stop you from using it. "We need to get over this myth that's floating around that only dry women use lubes," says Lori, adding that data indicates the vast majority of women use a lubricant. But if you're new to the lube game, she suggests buying one that's water-based and has a pump so you don't have to fiddle with caps, and keeping it on your bedside table for easy access. "Lube is a must every single time."

Hold up. Am I the only one who missed the memo on lube? Here I've been having sex without lube like an idiot, not realizing what I've been missing. After interviewing Lori, I was determined to find out—and fast.

Seconds after we spoke, I pulled up my Amazon app to research lubes. (Lest she who has not bought from Amazon cast the first stone.) I found many water-based options that, by the way, are safer than silicone- or oil-based lubes for both your body and your toys. Ultimately, I opted for the original, unscented lube from Lube Life, a brand with the optimistic motto "If you lube it, they will come." The 240 mL bottle did not have a pump but cost a reasonable $13.99, so I decided to buy it and deal with the cap.

Two days later, I opened the door to find the Amazon package on our front step. We couldn't wait to try our new tool, so while the kids watched a movie, we slipped away for a quickie in our room. Let me jump to the climax: Lube is glorious. It's silky smooth! It's so simple to use! It doesn't stain your sheets! And it makes orgasms more intense! No joke. The slippery substance is magical. We were doing the same things we always do, but everything felt smoother, better, more sensual.

Many months have passed since then, so you may be wondering: Have we kept up with the lube? Yes. Every. Single. Time. We even packed it for a quick trip to Mexico for a friend's wedding, so essential this lube had become only one month into our experiment. Me to Cam, before heading to the airport: "You have your passport? Shoes for the wedding? Lube?"

Side note: On our first day there, we forgot to put the bottle away before having our hotel room cleaned. We came back to find Lube Life sitting where the cleaners had placed it on the bedside table. For a hot second, we were mortified. Cam was convinced that word would spread and, by sundown, we'd be known by the hotel staff as The Lubies.

Whatever. I realized, I didn't even care. Let them know we use lube. We're not ashamed! May they be so lucky as to be lubies themselves.

I've come a long way since feeling embarrassed in that hotel room. In fact, I've undertaken a personal mission to bring up lube with my closest friends; most haven't been using it, but after I tell them about Lori's advice and my endorsement, they're eager to try. No doubt everyone who gives it a whirl will have a different experience, but I hope you feel curious enough to grab a bottle. And if you already have lube in your life, well done, you.

As someone who never thought I needed or would benefit from using lube, discovering its goodness has been nothing short of a revelation. Whether we're having maintenance-style sex or a more indulgent session, the lube adds a certain *je ne sais quoi* to the encounter. I will never go without it again.

Of all Lori's advice, introducing lubrication to my sex life yielded the most immediate results. The others were a slower burn but no less worth the effort. Because Cam and I already communicate well and plan sex, albeit loosely—we chat about the best times over the coming day or two, and we're good about booking date nights and the odd weekend away—I decided to focus on Lori's other tips: learning to stay present in my body and cultivating desire in between sexual encounters. These are strategies that can benefit every woman, regardless of your relationship status or how often you're having sex.

To improve my mind-body connection, I decided to give meditation a shot. With both Karen and Lori advocating for mindfulness to improve sex, I couldn't avoid it any longer. And believe me, I tried. I've never loved the idea of meditating, likely because I'm so bad at it. My mind is busy, and she does *not* want to be quieted. Plus, my daily to-do list is so long that finding time to sit, be still, and do nothing seems like a waste of precious time. But I know that logic is not sound. In fact, it's plain wrong.

Among many other benefits, meditation has been proven to help people reduce stress and anxiety, improve self-awareness and emotional regulation, sleep better, and tame racing thoughts. And as Lori shared, learning to stay more present can ultimately improve your ability to feel arousal and pleasure.

Hearing all this, I knew it was time to get over my aversion to meditation, dig in, and give it my best shot. First, I downloaded Insight Timer, a free, expert-recommended app. Next, buoyed by my tips from Dr. Russ Poldrack about how to make new habits stick (see chapter 7), I set a daily reminder on my phone to meditate. I even added the pink heart emoji so it would look cute and fun, not dull and snoozy.

Although, snoozy is exactly how I felt after completing the first session in the app's seven-day introduction to meditation series. During those ten minutes, though my thoughts were popping like popcorn kernels, I kept returning to my breathing to quiet my mind. It wasn't perfect, but the coach reminded me that's normal. I settled into a relaxing, calming breathing rhythm, and the chill feeling that came over me during the lesson stuck around for the rest of my workday.

I have been meditating for eight months now, and though I don't manage to swing it every day, it's become a habit I look forward to. Somewhere along the way I stopped viewing the daily practice as a task I must check off my to-do list and embraced it as a brief, lovely reprieve from whatever I'm worried about or stressing over. That said, three things have contributed to my success in keeping up with my new habit:

1. Having a daily reminder on my phone to make time for the practice, even if I must meditate before or after I had planned.
2. Setting a small, doable goal that isn't daunting or too time-consuming. For me, that means aiming to spend ten minutes a day meditating.
3. Looking forward to how great I will feel at the end of those ten minutes. On days I feel frantic, I remind myself how beneficial meditation is to my well-being and how much more centered I will be afterward.

After many months of practice, I'm seeing progress. It's much easier for me to quiet my thoughts, settle into deep breathing, and feel sensations and emotions in my body I would typically ignore.

That applies while I'm meditating and even when I'm not. If I'm worried or anxious, I will close my eyes and breathe into every part of my body, focusing on the areas I clench when I'm stressed: my shoulders and stomach. The stomach is a strange one, hey? Meditation helped me discover my tendency to tense my stomach muscles when I'm anxious. And having that awareness helps me to relieve the stress there.

But has improved mindfulness led to stronger desire and better sex? I mean, meditating isn't making me hornier by any means, but my meditation muscle, as I think of it, comes in handy during sex—and anytime I want to quiet my brain, really. For example, I often use a two-word phrase I picked up during my learn-to-meditate series: Not now. When I have unwanted or distracting thoughts pop up during foreplay or sex, I tell those thoughts, "Not now." It's simple. It helps. And it's much easier to stop thoughts from spiraling than before I started to meditate, a skill I'm grateful to have at the ready.

As for using the time in between sexual encounters to cultivate desire, well, that has been a ride. A scintillating, valuable ride.

And it all started with a book.

When one of my favorite bloggers, Lainey Lui from Lainey Gossip.com, wrote about a book called *The Idea of You* by Robinne Lee, I decided to buy it. The story is about a woman named Solène, a nearly 40-year-old mother who takes her daughter to see the girl's favorite boy band. When Solène ends up in a sexual relationship with the 20-year-old lead singer, Hayes, hot sex ensues.

Obvious comparisons to Olivia Wilde and Harry Styles aside, the book sounded light and different from my usual reads. I had never sought or bought a book for its sexy content before—a big mistake, in hindsight—so *The Idea of You* seemed like the perfect entry point. As Lainey wrote, "This is a very horny story . . . but it's more than just hot f-cking (although the f-cking is indeed very hot). This is also a story about a woman approaching midlife, giving herself permission to surrender to impulse, to take up space, to be the main character, to be the desired character."

For all those reasons, I loved the book. Not only was the story compelling and the writing solid, but the sex scenes felt realistic, intense, and not cringe-y at all. My whole body was lit up while I read them, and much like meditation's effects, that fiery feeling lingered well after I'd put the book down. Best of all, that feeling turned into action. My desire was so amped that I initiated sex more than usual and felt spicier in the sheets. All thanks to words on a page.

And here I've been reading regular books like an idiot, not even realizing what I've been missing.

I had just finished *The Idea of You* before interviewing Lori, so when she mentioned reading erotica can help ignite the body, I nodded in agreement. I had only dipped my toe into a sea of sexy content and was excited to dive in.

To continue my exploration of the wide world of erotica, I signed up for a free trial of Dipsea, a paid app offering an array of sexy audio stories. A friend of mine told me about it after I recommended *The Idea of You*, saying it helps her get in the mood. I downloaded the app, picked my turn-ons from their menu (sorry, those are between Dipsea and me), and voilà! Curated, sexy stories at my fingertips.

I'll admit, my first try felt odd. I'm not used to hearing other people talk dirty to each other, fool around, and even climax. It seemed like I was intruding. Or maybe it was weird because my kids were running around the house, and I was in the bathroom listening to the story with my Beats Fit Pro. Rookie mistake.

My second experience was slightly better. All alone at the end of the workday, I put Dipsea on our speakers and listened to a story while slicing veggies for dinner. (I ran outside not once but twice to make sure I wasn't accidentally broadcasting it over our outdoor speakers and turning on our neighbors.) The story itself was great, but listening while prepping dinner still didn't fire anything up but my oven.

I had no one to blame but me.

As Lori mentioned, no tool will be effective unless you focus on turning on your mind while you're using it. I was distracted when I tried the app—nothing screams turn-on like food prep—so I vowed to give it another try. When I was alone one afternoon, I ran a bath, lit a candle, cued the story up on my bathroom speaker, and settled into the tub. This time, the conditions were right. I enjoyed the story much more and paid attention to my body as I listened.

Still, on a turn-on scale of one to ten, I hit a lukewarm four.

When my free trial was up and I considered the app's annual fee of $79.99, I decided not to subscribe. For me, reading erotica seems more effective than listening to it. Plus, I could put that money toward a whole pile of books. I've since read another book that was steamy but not quite my jam, and I have another few books on hand to try, but I may give *The Idea of You* another spin first. That book hit all the right notes for me.

You know what else hits all the right notes for me? The discovery I mentioned earlier. (I wouldn't leave you hanging.) It's a sex toy, a vibrating ring you can use on your own or with a partner. It's a delight, is what it is. When worn around a penis, the We-Vibe Pivot is designed to fit between both partners during sex, but it's also excellent for solo play and foreplay. We're fans.

Disclaimer: Landing on a toy you love might take trial and error. We invested in some flops, like the We-Vibe Wand, a massive tool that vibrates, comes with two attachments, and made me feel like I was operating heavy machinery. Other people love it, though. As one reviewer wrote on we-vibe.com, "Pretty sure I cried rainbows and unicorns after the first 3 uses. Then waited a few minutes to come back to life. Try it."

I did, and I'll be sticking to smutty books and the Pivot, thanks.

Ultimately, what gives me pleasure and turns me on is just that—nothing but my pleasures and turn-ons. What are yours?

If you're not sure, midlife is an excellent time to find out.

"Our bodies are changing—they're changing all the time—so what our bodies like to experience is different," Karen says. "If you experience orgasms, what do your orgasms feel like? What parts of your body feel different? There's a lot of newness to be explored."

Newness. Renewal. Exploration.

These are words you don't typically hear when talking about sex for women over 40—and that's why I love them. The sexual goddesses within us are alive and well. They may just need a nudge to experiment and the permission to evolve.

Through my own experimentation, I've realized the key to better sex at this age is not finding time to have *more* of it. The key, for me, is twofold: making the most of each encounter and using the time in between sexual encounters to boost my desire, improve mindfulness, and become more comfortable in my body.

It's a constant evolution. And as I let go of the expectations I used to have for my body and sex life, I see the glimmers of a new sexual being emerging. She is confident. Joyful. And she loves a sexy book.

My hope is that each of us feels empowered to explore what brings us pleasure and embrace this stage of our sexual journeys. And the next one. And the one after that. Because when I look ahead to my late forties and beyond, what excites me most is knowing there will always be newness to explore. How exactly will my future sexual eras unfold?

I'm not sure, but I'll tell you this much: There will be lube.

THE CHEAT SHEET

- Be curious about self-stimulation, and if you're into it, embrace masturbation. Just like exercising or eating well, masturbating is part of a well-rounded health routine.

- Broaden your definition of pleasure. Any activity that makes you feel alive and connects you to a pleasurable sensation is worth pursuing.
- Spend a bit of time daily on a mindfulness practice of your choice. Learning to quiet the mind and stay present in your body will lead to better, more pleasurable sex.
- If you're in a relationship, talk about sex and don't be shy about planning it days, weeks, and even months ahead. Strong communication is the biggest predictor of long-term sexual satisfaction.
- Understand that, for women, pleasure often leads to desire, not the other way around. Suggest sharing small pleasures with your partner to see if desire kicks in from there, but don't feel badly if it doesn't.
- Always use a lubricant, whether for touch, sex, or anything else, because it will increase pleasure and ultimately boost desire. Look for a water-based lube with a pump and keep it on your bedside table for easy access.
- Read, watch, or listen to sexy content—whatever floats your boat and tingles your genitals. Foreplay starts when your last sexual encounter ends, so use the time in between to stoke your erotic fire.

CHAPTER TEN

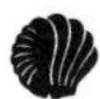

Achieve Maximum Sophistication with Simple Life Hacks

AT THIS POINT IN OUR ADULT LIVES, WE'RE EXPECTED TO KNOW adult things. For example, how to find art that's not from IKEA, invest our money to set us up for old age, spot a killer glass of wine on a menu, cook a meal for a group, build our wardrobes like a grown-up, and say the right thing to a loved one who's grieving. But how many of us gals know how to do all this? A better question might be: How many of us are willing to admit we don't know?

Don't fret, because in this chapter I have you covered. To help us achieve a life of maximum satisfaction and sophistication (or at least appear that way), I've talked to a wide array of experts to get the advice we need. I've been lucky to interview a few of these gals before, while others I hunted down specifically for their unique brands of genius. These experts can help us nail aspects of our lives that may seem trivial but are critical to our self-esteem, relationships, and futures.

And their advice works. I can attest that every tip, trick, and insight I gleaned from these accomplished women has improved my skill set, no matter the subject area. We have many how-to tips to cover, so let's start with a topic that never fails to excite me: food.

Make a One-Pot Meal to Wow Your Guests

Whether she's working with chefs at her restaurants, analyzing dishes in her role as resident judge on "Top Chef Canada," or whipping up food in her kitchen for family and friends, Janet Zuccarini is passionate about incredible food. As the founding CEO of Gusto 54 Restaurant Group, she has established award-winning restaurants in Los Angeles and Toronto beloved by celebrities and foodies alike.

I've been lucky to eat at a few of her restaurants, including her Los Angeles–based Italian eatery Felix. Soon after it opened in 2017, *Esquire* named Felix the #1 Best New Restaurant in America, and *Eater LA* dubbed it Restaurant of the Year. And, if anyone cares, Michelle McIvor calls her experience there The Best Meal of Her Life. I still dream about the pasta, bread, vibe, and stunning room. It's one of those meals I would happily relive repeatedly. Sadly, I don't live in Los Angeles. Happily, I have a friend who was willing to connect me with Janet. (Thank you, Rida!)

Janet and I spoke in the fall of 2022 about food, yes, but also about aging. Before we get to her recipe and hacks, I want to share a few of her thoughts because I found her outlook and zest for life inspiring.

At the time of our phone conversation, Janet was 57. She had just wrapped up an hours-long tennis match—a sport she learned to play only at 50. As someone who never considered herself an athlete, she was thrilled to discover a sport that excites her to get out of bed every morning. She says, "Tennis has turned into a massive passion."

Janet plays hours of tennis every day of the week—and plays it well. Three weeks before our call, she and her teammate competed nationally after winning their southern California division. "It was a tremendous experience," she says. "I didn't know I could become passionate about a sport, but it is my greatest joy."

Tennis is one of the reasons Janet says she's in better shape in her late fifties than she was in her twenties. She also prioritizes getting outside in the sunshine to walk or hike, and she follows the 80/20 guideline for eating nutritiously but indulging often. "I drink wine every single night. I eat gelato every single night," she says. "But I keep it all in check, and I do a lot to take care of myself. I feel like if you take care of your instrument, you'll play it for a long time."

I love that insight.

Because Janet feels better than ever at 57, I asked what advice she'd share with women younger than her. "Stop wasting your time worrying about aging. The bottom line is you're lucky," she says, "and if you've got your health, you have everything to enjoy this moment."

Spoken like a goddess.

I asked Janet to share a dish she makes when entertaining a large group. "I love making a one-pot meal for having family over, and they rave about this Tuscan chickpea and lacinato kale stew, also known as *Ribollita* in Italian," she says.

Buon appetito!

Ribollita (Tuscan Bean Soup)
Prep Time: 15 mins
Cook Time: 50 mins
Yields: 6–8 servings

Ingredients

⅛ cup good olive oil
½ cup chopped pancetta or bacon—optional (feel free to leave this out—or sub vegan bacon)
2 cups diced onions
1 cup diced carrots

(*continued*)

1 cup diced fennel bulb (or sub celery)
4–6 cloves garlic, rough chopped
1 tsp freshly ground black pepper
¼ tsp crushed red pepper flakes, or more to taste
2 tsp salt, plus more to taste
2–3 medium tomatoes, diced (or a 14-ounce can diced tomatoes)
6 cups lacinato kale, chopped
A splash of white wine
6 cups chicken or veggie stock
Parmesan rind (optional, but adds depth of flavor)
3 cups cooked cannellini beans (or use 2 cans cannellini beans, drained and rinsed, or great northern white beans)
½ cup chopped fresh Italian parsley leaves
Grated Pecorino or Parmesan (optional, or try vegan Parmesan)
Crusty bread

Rosemary Lemon Garlic Oil (for drizzling)

½ cup good olive oil
Zest of one large lemon
4 cloves garlic, sliced
A few sprigs rosemary (or thyme or sage)

Directions

1. Make the Rosemary Lemon Garlic Oil. Place all ingredients in a small jar or bowl and let sit on the counter (or make the day before, refrigerating overnight).

2. In a large, heavy-bottom pot or Dutch oven, heat oil over medium heat. Add onions and optional pancetta and sauté 6–8 minutes.
3. Lower heat to medium-low and add the carrots, fennel (or celery) and garlic, salt, pepper, and chili flakes, and cook another 7–9 minutes, until vegetables are tender.

4. Add the tomatoes and lacinato kale, and a splash of white wine, and continue sautéing and stirring occasionally for 7–8 minutes.
5. Add the stock and beans. Bring soup to boil, then turn heat down and simmer for 15 minutes. (You could add a Parmesan rind to the simmering soup for extra depth of flavor.)
6. Stir in fresh Italian parsley. Adjust salt if necessary. (If your soup is overly salty, see Janet's hack below!)
7. Serve in bowls with a drizzle of the flavorful lemon oil, grated Parmesan (or Romano), and crusty bread.

Janet's notes: If you like a thicker soup, blend or purée 1–2 cups of the soup, and add back to the soup. Or thicken it with day-old bread, torn into small pieces and cooked with the broth. This is the traditional way. (I prefer a brothier version of this soup, so I skip both and serve with toasty bread on the side instead.)

You can make the recipe vegan by using veggie broth and skipping the pancetta and cheese. The lemon oil will add a delicious flavor; I highly recommend it. Sometimes I'll add a tablespoon of nutritional yeast for a cheesier flavor and 1 tablespoon miso paste to add more depth. Up to you.

To make for a heartier meal, I will add buffalo mozzarella or ricotta and a dollop of pesto to the grilled crusty bread.

Last, if you have an overly salty soup or stew, be it when you make her recipe or another one, Janet recommends throwing in apple slices or potato slices to absorb the excess salt. Let them simmer for a while, remove them after they've absorbed some salt, and, voilà, enjoy your less-salty soup. She says this method is handy because you don't have to worry about adding more liquid or other ingredients to the pot to disperse the extra salt. Just remember not to overcook the potatoes; simmering the slices for about 30 minutes should do the trick.

Make a Nutritious No-Bake Chocolate Snack

When I need to have a snack and satisfy my sweet tooth (every single day at 3 p.m.), I turn to one person's recipes: Michelle McGrattan.

Michelle is a Toronto-based certified Precision Nutrition coach. And as you know if you read the introduction, for many years my go-to interviewee for all things nutrition was John Berardi, founder of the world-leading nutrition-coaching program Precision Nutrition. I trust John. I trust Michelle. And lucky for us, she agreed to contribute one of her all-star recipes for this book.

I've had the pleasure of interviewing Michelle before, and I so admire her ability to empower, inspire, and uplift women. On top of her nutrition coaching, she's a mom, fitness instructor, and creator of The Michelle Method, a program to help people be their best selves through fitness and nutrition. And I'm telling you right now: Her recipes are incredible.

On her website, themichellemethod.com, she shares many for free and offers digital cookbooks for download at affordable prices. I can vouch for *The Michelle Method E-Cookbook*, which is packed with recipes I turn to daily, from mini turkey meatloaf muffins for my lunches and the kale salad as a go-to side to her nutritious ninja muffins for my kids (spinach is the secret ingredient).

As for satisfying my daily craving with something sweet but nutritious, I love to have Michelle's Cookie Dough Cashew Protein Bars on hand. My husband loves them. My son loves them. My daughter won't touch them, but she won't touch 99.5 percent of foods.

These bars are simple to make, yummy, and healthy to boot. I mean, I don't want to tell you what to do with your life, but you should make this recipe ASAP.

Cookie Dough Cashew Protein Bars

Ingredients

1¼ cups oat flour
¼ cup almond flour
½ cup vanilla plant-based protein powder (Michelle also recommends Aphina Performance Protein Powder in the Toffee Coffee flavor, a vegan powder she formulated in partnership with Aphina, or another plant-based protein powder because it will set better than whey protein powder. You could sub whey, but the base will be stickier.)
¼ tsp Himalayan salt
¼ tsp baking soda
⅓ cup pure maple syrup
½ cup cashew butter
¼ cup unsweetened almond milk
1 tsp vanilla
½ cup chocolate chips
1 tbsp coconut oil
1 tbsp cashew butter

Directions

1. Line an 8×8-inch square baking dish with parchment paper.
2. Mix oat flour, almond flour, protein powder, salt, and baking soda in a large bowl.
3. Add in the maple syrup, cashew butter, almond milk, and vanilla. Stir until you have a large ball.
4. Using slightly wet hands or a baking spatula, press the dough evenly into the baking dish.

(*continued*)

5. Make chocolate coating by placing chocolate chips, coconut oil, and cashew butter in a small saucepan on low and stir until melted.
6. Pour the chocolate over the bars and use a spatula to spread evenly. Top with a sprinkle of Himalayan sea salt.
7. Freeze for 1–2 hours before slicing into 9 bars or 12 mini bars. Keep in an airtight container in the fridge or freezer. Enjoy!

A couple of my own notes: I'm allergic to cashews, so I use peanut butter instead of cashew butter and I opt for regular milk instead of almond milk (see chapter 1 for the background on why). Whichever way you decide to make them, these delicious, no-bake protein bars will boost your protein intake and satisfy your sweet tooth.

Improve Your Wellness with Three Doable Tips

When I connected with Dr. Krista Scott-Dixon, the former director of curriculum at Precision Nutrition mentioned in chapter 8, I intended to ask her about must-have nutrition tips for women in midlife. But the first moments of our call were a preview of a discussion that would encompass much more. Because when we jumped into our virtual chat room, Krista was . . . not still.

"Don't be alarmed," she told me. "I'm on a treadmill, in case you're wondering why I'm bobbing up and down."

Krista spends most of her workdays on the treadmill in her home office in Vancouver, writing emails, taking calls, and consulting with clients. She says it's how she does everything because she wouldn't do well sitting at a desk for eight hours. But it's more than that. As a woman in her forties who is striving to age with strength and independence, like her grandmother, Krista is a huge advocate for doing low-level, semi-constant, intermittent movement. Or, as she says, always finding ways to be in motion, like a shark that keeps swimming. It's what she encourages other women to do, too—often to their dismay.

"People think it's so unsexy and boring. Like, 'Oh great, a twenty-minute walk,'" she says. "We've become so fixated on burning calories. But every twenty-minute walk you take, or every time you take a flight of stairs, you're telling your body, 'Hey, we need tissue strength, we need stability, we need mitochondria.' It's the base of your iceberg that allows all the other things to happen."

I confess to thinking advice like this was boring when I was younger. Park as far from the mall entrance as you can and walk? Snooze. Always take the stairs? No thanks. But with age comes wisdom and knees that can't handle running. In the past few years, I've realized how good it feels to walk, an activity that doesn't stress my body too much but gets my blood pumping. I'll walk anywhere—to the corner store, through a park with a friend, around our neighborhood to get some fresh air. My body feels good after, and so does my mood. Like Krista, I encourage you to be a shark and see what happens.

She also had many other fantastic suggestions for women in midlife. Here are a few you can try, if not today, then soon:

- **Before investing in all kinds of supplements, get a simple blood test to determine your levels of vitamin D, iron, and B vitamins.** Krista recommends all women get their blood tested every now and then to see if they have the proper levels of essential vitamins and minerals. Whether you get one from a doctor or pay for one with a naturopath, checking your baseline before taking random supplements is a smart idea. "That way you're not randomly throwing things at the wall," she says. If you're lacking or low in something, supplement accordingly.
- **Get enough sleep.** Krista said it in chapter 8, but it's worth repeating: Sleep is the foundation for optimal well-being

and happiness. Set boundaries in your life to get enough sleep—seven hours minimum—every night. "Saying yes to sleep means saying no to other things, like work, volunteer commitments, even kids' activities," she says. "And that's hard, but you must be very intentional with your time and choose to prioritize sleep."

- **Ask yourself who you want to be when you're older and align your actions.** Krista says when women identify their values and priorities for aging, it's much easier to create sustainable, healthy habits to help them reach their goals. To do that, ask yourself who you are now, and who you want to be when you're 60 or 80. "Who's that amazing woman you want to become, and is what you're doing right now aligned with that?" asks Krista. "Spend your time and energy on things that are your true priorities."

Master Modern Etiquette

Myka Meier is the champion of modern-day etiquette for women. She's the two-time best-selling author of *Modern Etiquette Made Easy* and *Business Etiquette Made Easy* and the creator of a range of online finishing programs for women and teens. As she says on her website, mykameier.com, she is "absolutely not your grandmother's etiquette teacher."

I reached out to Myka to glean some of her top tips for women, be it to correct the faux pas we're inadvertently making, improve our confidence in social situations, or even choose the right email sign-off. Read on for an edited and condensed version of our email exchange. And get ready to refresh your email sign-off!

For women who aren't familiar with the idea, what is modern etiquette all about?

"Etiquette is simply this fabulous way to conduct ourselves to show others respect, kindness, and consideration in a situation! Adding the word modern is key to understanding and practicing etiquette, because as society evolves, etiquette must evolve with it . . . hence why I am passionate about teaching modern etiquette. To learn and practice modern etiquette will help you thrive in everyday business and social situations with ease."

And how can mastering etiquette improve our lives and relationships?

"Etiquette is far more than just which fork and knife to pick up. It is a way to communicate and connect with people. Sure, it's good etiquette to practice good table manners, but that is simply because we want to show the person we are dining with respect. Understanding and practicing good modern etiquette will make you more confident, likeable, and successful, because people want to socialize with, do business with, and spend time with people who know how to navigate any situation.

One example is walking into a room and knowing how to start a conversation with anyone, no matter how much or little you have in common, then how to keep a conversation going, and also how to introduce them to others and network so that everyone feels happy and comfortable. Gliding through any networking situation, be it a cocktail party or work event, allows you to be more successful in both your work and business lives."

My book is designed to give women practical, accessible tips to help them live, look, and feel better. On the "look" front, what are a few of your go-to tips for women who want to look polished and put together?

"It can be exhausting to try to look your best every day, especially while balancing so many life tasks and responsibilities. Therefore, try this trick instead—it's called the two-of-three rule. The three things are your outfit, your skin, and your hair. The guideline here is to make sure you have at least two of the three put together before you leave the house. So, if you are in something casual, spend time on your hair and skin. If your hair is not done, then balance it out with your outfit and skincare or makeup routine. It will help you look a bit more polished daily."

What's the one area you think women at this stage of life need the most help with when it comes to etiquette? And can you share a tip or two on how to quickly improve those skills?

"I think sometimes entering new social groups can be difficult. I genuinely think it goes back to basics, with being kind and open minded, learning to be brave and approach others, introducing yourself, being able to ask genuine questions to show engagement, and, finally, following up. Sometimes you have to get out of your comfort zone, mentally prepare, knock any self-consciousness on its head, and come ready!

Try preparing yourself with a technique from my book *Modern Etiquette Made Easy*, which I call the 'back pocket three.' They are three questions or conversation topics—preplanned—that you're going to ask if the conversation runs out of steam: one newsworthy topic, one related to that event, and one local or current event you're interested in or knowledgeable about. It takes five minutes to think about them beforehand on your way to the event or meeting, and it's guaranteed you'll have something to pull out of your back pocket to talk about!"

In your opinion, which email sign-off should be abolished? And what's your go-to?

"It truly depends on the industry you are in. A trendy marketing firm's sign-off is likely completely different from a corporate bank's. My go-to is Best Regards when I want to be formal or corporate, and Warmest Regards if I want to come across softer."

What are the one or two etiquette mistakes you see women in midlife make that you wish you could fix for good?

"Not standing when they shake hands or introduce themselves. Many women in certain generations were taught not to stand and only that men should stand when meeting, greeting, or shaking hands. As I teach modern etiquette, I teach very genderless and give power and confidence through etiquette. No matter your gender, you should stand to shake hands or when introduced to show respect, confidence, and that you are empowered both in business and socially. I also think women should have a firm and assertive handshake to show confidence upon meeting."

Is there anything you are passionate about sharing with women that we haven't touched on?
"It's never too late to start learning etiquette. I only learned as an adult, and it changed my life. I also think every day is a new chance to make a first impression, so never forget that."

Last, how do you feel about aging?
"To me, it's simply graduating to the next level and moving on with more power under your wings. As we age, self-care is very important and sometimes [you may need to schedule] it into your calendar. Remember, it's not a luxury. It's a priority, ladies!"

Find, Buy, and Install Quality Art

Tamar Zenith knows good art. She's the co-director of Newzones Gallery of Contemporary Art, which she and her mother started together in Calgary in 1992. Since then, they've built Newzones into one of North America's leading contemporary art galleries. The gallery happens to be in my city—lucky for me because I'm in love with the art they promote. (Check it out at newzones.com, where you can browse pieces and request price information. They ship internationally, too.) My husband and I pop in every so often to check out their collections and daydream about which artist we'll choose the next time we add a quality piece to our collection.

We're not aficionados, by any means, nor do we buy art often. But we enjoy hanging pieces in our home that speak to us somehow. Over the last eight years, we've acquired one painting from a gallerist, commissioned another from a local artist, shipped a large print from a Los Angeles–based photographer and framed it upon arrival, and ordered a painting from UGallery.com, a site connecting artists directly with buyers. But we've also found many affordable pieces at the Alberta University of the Arts' Show + Sale, an event featuring the work of students who are up-and-coming artists.

Ultimately, though, we have no rhyme or reason to choosing our art. We've just gone with what makes us feel good.

According to Tamar, that's a decent strategy! Over coffee on a sunny day in June 2023, I picked her brain about how to find, buy, and hang art, because having that kind of skill set feels chic.

So, if you're ready and excited to upgrade your art collection, read on for her top tips.

On finding art: "Always go to a reputable gallery. Start with ones accredited by the Art Dealers Association of Canada and the Art Dealers Association of America. Just like when you buy *anything* luxury, you want to make sure it has backing behind it—and to be part of those associations, there are criteria you have to meet. And even if a piece in my gallery is less expensive than others, you know the art has met *my* criteria. I want to promote it, place it, and I believe in the artist.

Also, go somewhere you feel welcome. It's nice to have a relationship with your dealer. That's how many of my great friendships have been made over the years because, obviously, if someone's walking in and interested, we have a commonality.

If you're interested in art, seek out galleries in the cities and areas you're visiting. Just like people seek out the best restaurants when they're traveling, seek out the best galleries. Explore, see what you like, and it might make you appreciate the galleries in your hometown more, too."

Follow-up: Find the Art Dealers Association of Canada at ad-ac.ca and the Art Dealers Association of America at artdealers.org to find galleries near you or wherever your travels take you.

On choosing a piece: "You just have to love it. We always say, 'Your couch is going to change. Your walls are going to change. But if you have a piece that moves you, you're always going to love it and it will look good wherever.'

And if you can start with a price point or budget you're comfortable with, a gallerist will be happy to figure out a way that works for you. At my gallery, for example, we offer young collectors an interest-free payment plan to make buying art as easy as possible because we want the artists and their pieces out there."

Pro tip: Ask the galleries with artwork you love if they offer payment plans, ideally with zero interest, for their customers.

On installing art: "People love to hang their art high, but it should be at eye level. I think some people worry their kids will do stuff to their art, but your kids aren't taking colors to your car! You just have to let them know.

At our gallery, we install at 52 inches center, meaning the center of the piece is 52 inches from the floor. Some people do 57 inches, but to me that appears a little bit high. Here's the basic formula: Measure the height of the piece in inches and divide it by two; from that number, subtract the number of inches between the top of the frame and the D rings or whatever the work will hang from; then add 52. The final number is the height in inches, measured from the floor, telling you where to put the hangers or hooks into the wall."

Homework: Measure from the floor to the center of a piece of art or two hanging in your home to see how you've fared. Don't worry. You can always rehang art! Plus, every situation is a little different, says Tamar. Depending on your furniture height and other factors, you may need to install higher or lower than 52 inches.

Build Your Wardrobe Like a Grown-up

As a long-time fashion expert, stylist, costume designer, and wardrobe buyer for shows and movies such as "The Last of Us" and "Ghostbusters: Afterlife," Crystal Mckenzie has seen more than a few trends come and go—and then come back again. So she heeds a simple rule and encourages her clients to do the same: "Wear whatever makes you happy."

For Crystal, whom I have the pleasure of bumping into now and then in our shared city of Calgary, the pieces that make her happy are designer bags and statement glasses. "But style is a very individual thing," she says. "There are no specific, perfect pieces any woman needs. It's about wearing whatever makes you feel great and gives you confidence."

But there *is* one strategy she recommends for women in midlife interested in building or broadening their wardrobes. "At this age when your career is more established, and you likely have more income flowing, invest in the high-quality pieces that will last a lifetime," she says. Choose quality over quantity to invest in what you love—a well-fitted blazer, the perfect white dress shirt, or a great pair of jeans. Because whether you buy new, from a consignment store, or second-hand, spending more on items that make you feel confident, happy, and fabulous will be worth it. "How you dress is how you're perceived in the world," Crystal says. "Have fun with it because there are many ways to look cool."

Order, Buy, and Enjoy Wine Like a Pro

Bianca Bosker's bestselling book *Cork Dork: A Wine-Fueled Adventure Among the Obsessive Sommeliers, Big Bottle Hunters, and Rogue Scientists Who Taught Me to Live for Taste* taught me many things about wine. But one tip forever changed how I choose a glass of wine at a restaurant or bar. The strategy is simple: I pick the glass I don't recognize. Be it wine from a region I don't know or made with a grape I'm unfamiliar with, I go for it.

Why? According to Bianca, who left her job as a technology reporter to become a sommelier and write about her experiences, there's a logic that sommeliers use to build a by-the-glass wine list—and it's often in your best interest to order the glass you don't recognize. That's because sommeliers often charge a premium for the glasses people are most familiar with and automatically order, no matter the price. Think the Sauvignon Blancs, Cabernet Sauvignons, Chardonnays, Pinot Grigios, and Merlots of the world. Order any of those glasses and you may not get the best bang for your wine-loving buck.

On the other hand, when you see a wine you're unfamiliar with, it's there because someone else is passionate about it and wants to share it with others. To encourage more people to take a risk on *those* glasses, sommeliers will price them lower—meaning you're likely to get a high-quality wine for good value.

That gem of an insight has stuck with me since I read *Cork Dork* six years ago and led to me discover all kinds of wines I enjoy and would order again. I had the chance to thank Bianca when we connected for a chat on Christmas Eve in 2022, a conversation I couldn't wait to have because I'm such a fan of her work.

Read on for our (edited and condensed) Q and A about all things wine, from what Bianca's drinking lately to how she chooses a bottle for a dinner party and more. And prepare to never pick a bottle of vino the same way again.

First, I must tell you: I loved your tip about how to order wine at a restaurant and use it all the time.

"Yes, the by-the-glass list! What I learned about the hidden logic of that list is there are these 'gimme' wines, which are the ones people instantly recognize and say, 'I know what that is. Gimme a glass of that. I don't care how much it costs.' So people can charge more for those, at least in my experience. I can't say this is true for every restaurant, but the wines on the list from a wine region you've never heard of or a grape you can't pronounce are there because someone loved them."

We have discovered great wines thanks to that tip, so thank you! When you attend a dinner party these days, what wine do you bring?
"I worked for Paul Grieco, who runs Terroir, which is still one of my favorite places to drink wine in New York. And he would make people promise to never drink the same wine twice. When I first heard that, I thought that was ridiculous and absurd. And it took me a really long time to realize he's completely right. Of course, there are those bottles that we come back to again and again, and they change. You change. But it's like books. There are more books in the world than you could ever read in a lifetime. There are more wines than you could ever drink in a lifetime, so why not branch out and try something new?

I have really taken that advice to heart with my own drinking. When I'm serving wine for a dinner party at home or I'm bringing wine to someone's house, I think less about it being delicious—I *hope* it's delicious—but I think about it more as how I'm going to take people on a journey. Like, how is this bottle going to be an adventure? Especially when I'm at a restaurant picking wine. As you can imagine, if you've written a book about wine, there's a lot of pressure to not screw it up and to pick a good bottle of wine! The reality is I haven't tried every wine in the world. But when I don't recognize what's on the list or in a wine store, I try to pick a wine with something that excites me, whether it's a region I don't know or a grape by a producer I've never tried or from a part of the world I'm unfamiliar with. I don't play it safe, and that means often I'm not spending a ton of money because if the price is starting to hurt, it's hard to take risks.

I want to be able to tell people why this is an exciting adventure we're going to take, why this isn't just fermented grape juice we're going to drink. To me, that's what's so exciting about wine.

The pandemic really drove that home—that when you uncork a bottle of wine, you're uncorking the smells, the tastes, the flavors of a different period, of a different place on the planet. I love this idea that you can travel through space and time without ever leaving your seat, through a glass of wine."

Are you drawn more to white or red wine?

"I'm personally drawn more to white wines. There's been this meme around for a long time that red wine is for serious wine drinkers and that white or sweet wines are what you drink before you've matured into red wine. I don't buy any of that. It's a personal taste thing, but I'm here to tell people: If you like white wines, if you like sweet wines, if you like orange wines, like what you like!"

What tips are you passionate about sharing with people?

"There are a few skills that will help you a great deal in figuring out what you like and classifying the information in your head in a productive way. And I think the first piece of that is developing your sense memory. When we have a glass of wine in front of us, our first tendency is to put it in our mouth. And that's fine. That's what it's there for. But I think most of us—and this is true for me before I went on this whole journey to train as a somm—miss what has now become my favorite part of the wine, which is just smelling it.

We can pick up around five different tastes, where scientists argue that we can pick up something like a trillion odors. And so much of the nuance of a wine really is in its smell. So, there's nothing I would encourage doing more than smelling everything. I trained with sommeliers but also a master perfumer whose advice was to describe the smell of everything that I encountered during my daily life, from my shampoo in the morning to the black pepper I put on my dinner at night.

Smell is hard, but it gets easier over time. Most of us grow up learning the cow goes 'moo' and the grass is green, but we don't necessarily learn to identify the smell of lavender or strawberry. And you're never going to smell strawberry in a wine if you can't smell strawberry in a strawberry. That's why smelling things and putting words to the smells is a critical first step; it locks in the scents for us.

The Wine Aroma Wheel by Ann Noble is a great starting point because it has a library of smells that are very common in wine but are also things you can find in the supermarket. Smelling apple, orange, green bell pepper—that will help you train your nose."

I know you don't like to drink the same wine twice, but what have you been loving lately?

"It's been an ongoing love affair with white wines from northern Italy and Slovenia. There's some bias because my mother's family is from that area, but the Friuli Venezia Giulia region and Slovenia make some really great, interesting white wines. I do like orange wines, and I like to serve a lot of sparkling wines, like Champagne or other sparkling wines with different grapes from different regions, because I don't think they only have to be for festive occasions, and they pair nicely with just about anything you want to eat. Also whites from Sicily. Oh my God, there's something about a Grillo, a grape from Sicily, in the summertime. It's like a vacation in a bottle."

Any last advice to share?

"For someone who's trying to build up their wine expertise, it's helpful to start with the noble grape varieties—the ones that show up over and over again throughout the world, like Sauvignon Blanc, Cabernet Sauvignon, Pinot Noir, Chardonnay. There are others, too, but I suggest drinking only one, like Sauvignon Blanc, from different parts of the world for a month until you really understand the essence of Sauvignon Blanc. How is the one from France different from the one from New Zealand? And how is it similar? After that, drink only Chardonnay for a month. This is why it's good to get a tasting group or a group of friends to drink with—a bottle of wine is 750 milliliters and designed to be shared.

When you're drinking wine, I would also try to pick up two pieces of information about that bottle to begin to build your mental map. It could be what grape it's made with and where it's made. That can be helpful in orienting yourself. And there are apps you can use to keep track, or you could just make an emoji tasting note in your phone—doing anything that imprints your impression of that wine will help build your foundation."

Declutter Your Home to Destress Your Life

There's a reason we all feel great when we walk into a clean, organized hotel room, says Megan Golightly: We're inhabiting a calm, clutter-free zone where everything has its place. "You've brought a small amount of things that you could live with—you have your favorite clothes, your best book, your go-to toiletries," says Megan, owner of the Calgary-based personal organization company Simplified. And being unencumbered by our usual clutter is a freeing experience. "We all want to feel light. But because we're hunters and gatherers, we feel like we have to layer on more and more and more in our lives."

Through her work with Simplified, Megan has helped thousands of people across North America climb out from under their clutter, including former "Bachelorette" Jillian Harris, singer Jann Arden, and mega-influencer Sarah Nicole Landry, aka @thebirdspapaya. I first connected with Megan in 2022 to interview her for a magazine story I contributed to *Chatelaine*, one of Canada's top national publications for women, about how she worked with Sarah to organize her home in Guelph, Ontario. Most recently, we grabbed coffee to chat about her top tips for you, my dear readers. (Megan and I also live around the corner from each other—a lovely surprise when we found out!)

Not only is Megan a master declutterer, she uses her background in psychology and her interest in neuroscience to help people break through the psychological barriers holding them back from tackling their messiest areas. Decluttering may be hard when you start, but rest assured it's a skill that can be developed, honed, and maintained. And the effort is well worth it.

Here are a handful of the benefits to decluttering your living spaces, according to Megan:

- **You gain time.** Because you're not managing and navigating so many things in your home, you have more time to relax, be present, and enjoy your surroundings.
- **You save money.** When every area of your home is organized and you can see what you have on hand, such as pantry and bathroom supplies, you're not repurchasing items you already own.
- **Your relationships thrive.** Megan says many of her clients report having better relationships with their partners and kids after decluttering and organizing their homes because they're not bickering or fighting about mess and clutter.
- **Your mental and physical health improve.** There's a cost to clutter. "Women's cortisol goes up with clutter," Megan says, making us feel overwhelmed, stressed, and anxious. As she said for our *Chatelaine* story, "When you keep too many things, it becomes visual clutter, which turns into mental clutter."

Clutter isn't fun to look at, nor does it do our bodies or brains any favors. But we can defeat it—and we *will*, thanks to Megan's insights. Here are her top three tips on how to tackle your messiest areas:

1. **Don't even think about organizing your spaces before you declutter them.** Megan equates decluttering to having a learner's license, and organizing as the driver's license. You

need the former to move on to the latter. "You cannot organize without decluttering first, but we automatically jump to organizing," she says. "That's because decluttering is the psychologically hard part." Decluttering means getting rid of things that have not earned the right to be in your home, but letting go is hard. Megan points to common traps that people fall into when trying to discard, donate, or sell things, such as being scared of making the wrong decision, holding onto items for sentimental reasons, keeping goods just in case you might need them, carrying guilt about how much money you spent on something, and worrying you might not have enough to last you in the future. "It's human nature to fall into these traps," she says, "but you need to get out of your own way. It comes down to: How badly do you want this? If you're serious about decluttering, you need to get tough with your things."

2. **Ask yourself these three questions of each item: Do I love it? Do I use it? Would I buy it again today?** You'll know the answer right away, Megan says. Okay, within three seconds max. If it's not a hard yes, then it's a no—and you should get rid of the item. She says, "When you start asking those questions, you'll never look back."

3. **Start your decluttering journey in the bathroom.** While learning how to declutter, it's best to tackle a room where you're likely to succeed. "The easiest place to train your brain that you can declutter is your bathroom," Megan says. "It's small, there aren't many personal things in there, and it's easier to ask yourself those questions because you have fewer emotional triggers." Once you've conquered the bathroom, you can move on to trickier areas such as your master closet, garage, pantry, and storage room. "The sooner you get on it, the sooner you'll see you can live with less."

After you've successfully decluttered your bathroom (congrats—you've earned that learner's permit!), *then* you can begin to organize it—a process that will be much easier with less stuff to navigate. Megan offers many organizing tips for free on her Instagram account (find her at @gosimplified) and shares links to her favorite organizational items from stores like IKEA and Amazon. (I've bought a few of her recommendations, and my underwear and bra drawer has never been so tidy.) She also sells downloadable how-to guides on her website, go-simplified.com, with detailed instructions on organizing your home's messiest spaces, including the kitchen, pantry, office, and linen closet.

Before you check those out and move on to driver's license activities, I'll share an organizing tip from Megan that has revolutionized how we organize our pantry—and I suspect it would in yours, too: Decant your dry goods into clear, labelled containers. That means items like pasta, cereal, rice, flour, sugar, quinoa, coffee beans, and protein powder now live in clear, labelled containers in our pantry.

Decanting serves a few purposes, says Megan. It makes it easier to find what you're looking for and to spot when you're running low on something. It also eliminates the bulky, hard-to-store boxes and bags the goods came in. In their place is a row of neat, tidy containers, which thrill my inner organizational nerd every time I pull one out. For these reasons and more, I cannot recommend decanting enough.

But first, don't skip the critical step: Cut down on your clutter! Your house (and your brain) will thank you.

Start Building Your Wealth with These Three Tips

If the spending habits I've mentioned in the previous chapters haven't given it away, I'm not exactly frugal. Nor have I spent much time managing my money lately. That's because my husband is a chartered financial analyst who loves taking care of our investments. Before we were married, though, I managed to get my financial ducks in a row by myself. Sort of. I credit the investment advisor who helped guide my decisions when I started to make more money. All I did was implement his advice.

Having experienced how beneficial the right advisor can be, I decided to enlist an expert to share her insights into what you should look for when seeking a wealth advisor and how we can all begin to build wealth faster and prepare ourselves for the future. Enter Julie Shipley-Strickland, a Calgary-based senior wealth advisor with Wellington-Altus Private Wealth and an insurance advisor through Strickland Financial Group Ltd. In her own words, she's an entrepreneur passionate about connecting with people on their wealth on a human, warm level. "Wealth is a very cold, formal, stiff subject for most people," she says. "I want to add warmth and a real essence of humanity."

When I asked Julie to share her advice for women interested in creating a healthier financial future for themselves, she had three top tips:

1. **Just start saving.** "It sounds ridiculous, but in the wealth-building realm, you need to just start," Julie says. If you don't have a savings account yet earmarked for your retirement, now is the time to head out and open one! In Canada, your options include a Registered Retirement Savings Plan or a Tax-Free Savings Account. In the United States, investors have access to traditional and Roth Individual Retirement Accounts and 401(k) retirement plans, among others. Not sure which one you need? Proceed to step 2.

2. **Get credible advice from a qualified person.** On any given day, you'll find loads of wealth-building advice circulating online and on social media platforms like TikTok and Instagram. Julie's tip: Proceed with caution. "I see some advice and think, 'That is blatantly wrong!'" she says. "Getting credible information from someone who's living,

working, and breathing investment advice is key." Here's what to look for: a license or certification, such as the Certified Financial Planner® designation, indicating in-depth knowledge of financial planning for individuals; experience showing a track record of client success; and someone who, ideally, is personally invested in your success. In Julie's case, for example, part of her compensation depends on how her clients' money performs. If it increases, she is rewarded, and vice versa. That's not how it works with many advisors at banks, where employees get paid no matter what happens with your portfolio. Last, Julie suggests finding someone who really cares about your goals and shares in your excitement to save for the future. "There are a lot of different advisors out there, so you need to find a solution that works best for you."

3. **Take the amount you're comfortable saving and stretch it a bit more.** For example, if you're comfortable saving $500 a month right now, start saving $550. Or if you're comfortable saving $100, bump it to $125. "You're not really going to miss the $25, but the impact on your portfolio magnified over thirty or forty years will be massive because of compound interest," she says. Stretching how much you save every month, however small, is an effective strategy for anyone who's starting out. Julie says, "It's minimal impact to your bottom line right now, maximum impact for retirement."

Comfort Someone Who's Grieving

If you've ever wondered what to say to someone grieving, you're not alone.

It's not always easy finding the words to comfort someone who's lost a loved one, a job, or a pet, or is weathering a difficult life event like divorce. For advice on how to say and do the right thing when someone you know is in crisis mode, I called upon Dr. Susan Silk, a clinical psychologist based in Southfield, Michigan. Why Susan? Because I've relied on her advice since April 2013, when she and her husband, Barry Goldman, contributed an article to the *Los Angeles Times* in which she shared her now-famous "Ring Theory."

Susan told me their article is the most-viewed article the *Times* has ever run, which doesn't surprise me; no one knows what to say in a crisis, and her advice is brilliant. But despite its popularity, Susan doesn't have a fancy laminated or framed copy of the Ring Theory in her office. She still draws it on a piece of yellow paper when working with patients.

Here's how it can work for you in a crisis or trauma situation. First, draw a ring. In this ring, write the name of the person in crisis. It could be you or someone you know. Next, draw a larger circle around the middle ring and write the names of people next closest to the crisis, like a significant other or kids. Keep repeating this process, using the next larger rings for the next

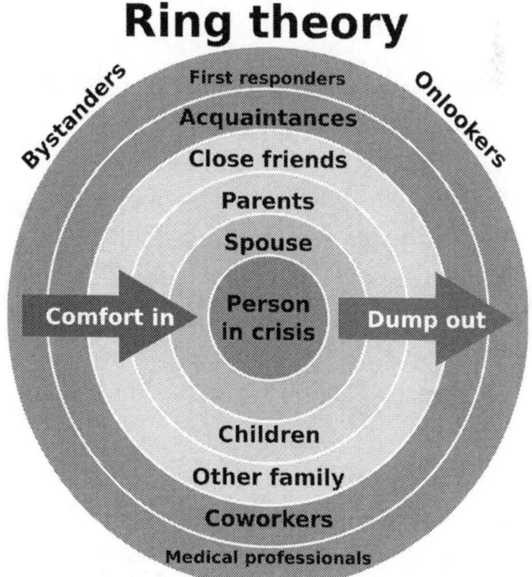

SOURCE: VALEREEE, CC BY-SA 4.0, VIA WIKIMEDIA COMMONS.

closest people. As Susan and Barry wrote, "Parents and children before more distant relatives. Intimate friends in smaller rings, less intimate friends in larger ones. When you are done, you have a kvetching order."

As for the Ring Theory in action, if you're in the center ring, you can say anything to anyone, anytime. You have carte blanche to complain, worry, whine, and bitch. If you're not in the center ring, you can still do all of that, too, but only to people in rings larger than yours. This behavior upholds the Ring Theory's core advice: Comfort IN, dump OUT.

But how do we comfort someone well? That's what I wanted to ask Susan.

Yet again, her wisdom was brilliant. Without further ado, here's how she recommends comforting someone weathering a crisis or going through a stressful live event:

- **First and foremost, be a good listener.** "Make yourself available and be a good listener," Susan says. That means resisting the urge to chime in with advice or a story of your own about a similar experience. For example, when somebody talks about their divorce, don't talk about yours. If their pet died, don't relate it to when your pet died. This is their moment, and your primary role is to listen. "It's great that we all have that instinct to help, and we don't want to shame people about that, but we ought to think, 'Is what I'm about to say really likely to help in this moment?'" To put this advice into practice, Susan suggests using a strategy from Alcoholics Anonymous, the acronym WAIT, which stands for Why Am I Talking? If you listen well and keep WAIT in mind, you'll show up well for someone in distress.
- **Stick to the tried-and-true "I am so sorry."** It sounds corny and like it might not be useful, says Susan, but saying, "I am so sorry"—even if you keep repeating it—is your

best bet. You can also say, "This must be so hard." Whether you say it in person, write it in a card, or send it in an email, your (brief) words will be appreciated.

- **Don't ask how you can help. Instead, offer choices.** Rather than saying, "Let me know if there's something I can do to help," which isn't actually helpful and places the burden of asking for help on the person in crisis, Susan suggests sharing a few specific ways you can help and letting them choose one. For instance, you could say, "I can drop off a macaroni-and-cheese casserole, swing by the hospital with coffee and snacks, or shovel your sidewalk. Let me know which one you want." The other option is to just act, performing an act of service without asking. And if you're not in the same city, get creative. You can send cards, flowers, or gift cards for food delivery services to show you care.

Last, we should cut ourselves some slack if, in retrospect, we did a poor job of supporting someone in their time of need. Susan uses a wedding as an example. If you realize you added stress to your friend's big day or somehow made it about you—perhaps dumping IN instead of OUT—that's okay. We're all human. But don't pretend it didn't happen. Susan advises, "You can say to your friend with humor, 'Oh my God, you were going through something, and I made it about me. I'm sorry. I can't believe I did that.' I think that's so corrective in a friendship."

CHAPTER ELEVEN

Age with Pride

Growing up, I was lucky to be surrounded by women who made aging look amazing.

My dad's mother, Florence, swam laps every morning, cross-country skied every winter, created gorgeous pottery, square-danced with my grandpa, and sewed stunning outfits, among other interests and hobbies. She once told me that life is a "forever adjust," a motto my husband and I often repeat.

My mom's mother, Adaliane, was no different. She was an incredible golfer and curler, dominated at bridge tournaments, and loved a good word game, not to mention a great party. She traveled the world with my grandfather and, even after he died, kept exploring with my uncle, aunt, and mom.

And, of course, my mother, the woman I look up to like no other. After taking years off work when my brother and I were young, she returned to teaching high school French. I have always admired her for pursuing a career she loved while raising a family, seeing friends, and tackling activities like aerobics and racquet sports. These days, she's vibrant as ever in retirement, prioritizing time with friends and family, enjoying symphony and theater performances with my dad, and spending time at our family cabin.

Whether they've known it or not, the women in my family have inspired me not to fear aging, to embrace every stage and age with pride. Having their examples to guide the way has been invaluable, so I set out to find us a few more.

I found them, and I can't wait for you to read their thoughts.

The following three women are not only accepting aging, they're pro-aging. Chatting with them lit me up and cemented my own status as a pro-aging gal. In sharing our conversations, which I have condensed and edited for your reading ease, I hope they make you feel excited for the next chapter of your journey, too.

Helen Tansey

Helen Tansey is a sought-after Toronto-based photographer and the host of the Coming into Focus podcast, a space she created to change how we view aging. In her late fifties herself, she believes aging is not something to hide or fix. Helen says getting older is a gift and that it does not take away from her value—it increases it. And she's determined to help inspire others feel the same.

In 2019, Helen published *Sundari Women*, a coffee-table book featuring her black-and-white portraits of women between ages 40 and 96, accompanied by each woman's thoughts on aging. *Sundari* means "beautiful" in Sanskrit, and Helen is passionate about capturing women's raw, natural beauty. Her book is an ode to women, a celebration of their strength, wisdom, and beauty as they age, and a defiant stance against the narrative that older women become invisible, small, and irrelevant. "Being a woman and getting older is a privilege," she wrote in the foreword. "Let's inspire others and ourselves by embracing this power and privilege every day. Time is on our side. We are not invisible. We are vibrant, glorious goddesses who deserve to be celebrated at every stage of our magnificent lives."

I was thrilled when Helen agreed to meet in person and chat about her take on aging—and floored when she offered to take my author photo for this book, and so very grateful. We met at her studio on a sunny day in May 2023 to get it all done. What follows are highlights from our lovely conversation.

Can you tell me about what inspired you to create your book?
"I tend to specialize in photographing actors, but as I have grown as a woman, my business has grown with me. When I was interested in having kids, I photographed more pregnant women. I always found them so beautiful. And then, when I had my boys, I started taking more pictures of kids. But in my forties, I didn't like the message about aging as a woman. Older women were not being represented in a positive light, and it really bothered me.

I knew I wanted to do something but didn't know what until my early fifties, when I started taking pictures of beautiful women of all ages and having them share their wisdom. I turned that into *Sundari Women*, and, in a way, it's my legacy. I wanted to leave something for my boys, who are now 17 and 19, to help them look at women in a positive light, to not only see women's age or have limited beliefs about what's possible for them."

Where does your appreciation for aging come from?
"I never feared getting older. When I looked at my mom, her friends, even older women on the bus, I actually couldn't wait to get older. And I think because I lost my brother at a young age, I realize how fortunate we are to be here. He didn't get to realize his dreams, but we still can. I'm 57 and don't want to feel like the best of my life is behind me. I still want to dream, to go after things and achieve them. I want to age in a way that is expansive.

Aging is hard sometimes, though, and I think a lot of it has to do with the messaging that getting older means doors are shutting or we're 'less than' because we have gray hair and wrinkles. We can change that messaging so women feel good about getting older. We are so much more than what we look like, but it is hard to break free of that."

Given you started your career as a model, I can imagine that's tough, especially when you're likely judged more harshly than other women. How do you break free of the expectations about how you should or shouldn't be aging?

"First of all, when I was younger, I never looked at myself and saw beauty. These days, if I start focusing on my looks or weight, I know something else in my life is off. Because when I feel good about myself, I can have dirty hair and wear sweatpants and feel like a million dollars. Part of aging is letting go and not attaching to an idea of what you were or how you were and just being present for who you are right now. And it's easier said than done, but I practice, and when I'm hard on myself, I ask why and look at what's triggering that feeling."

What does your self-care routine look like?

"I practice Buddhism, and having a healthy meditation practice helps me. It's my non-negotiable. Every morning after waking up, I take my dog out and then start my practice, which is usually an hour long and includes some Buddhist chants and journaling. I also eat well and drink lots of water. Well, that's a lie. I need to drink more water! And then I just try to enjoy my life. I love my boys. I love my husband. They bring me so much joy."

I have a 5-year-old daughter and a 7-year-old son, and I want to raise them to feel good about themselves, their bodies, and their age. Do you talk to your boys much about aging?

"I think integration between younger and older people is important. Even when we visit my mother or mother-in-law, my boys see aging and know it's not this taboo subject or something to fear. And it extends beyond family. I have friends that are my age, I have friends in their seventies, and I have friends in their thirties. I love that! I've learned a lot from my girlfriends, no matter their age, and they've learned from me. I don't think we should just stick to our clan."

When you look ahead to your next chapter, what excites you most?
"One of the beautiful things about aging is we have the money to travel because we've been working for a while. I love traveling, so if I want to go to Costa Rica or back to Maui to surf, I can do that. And when I think about retiring, why would I? People still want to work with me, and I'm enjoying it.

I still have so much passion and things I want to do, like the series I'm doing right now with my photography called 'Mother.' As mothers, there are all these invisible strings to our children and things we do behind the scenes. I don't know if I'll do a book again, but I love celebrating women. And I want to do more of my podcast to support women so that we can feel good about ourselves as we age and even feel excited about it. Because when I'm around women who own it—I don't care what age they are—and they're comfortable in their skin, I am so excited.

Also, as I get older, I enjoy more time to myself. I love having tea, journaling, and doing my own thing. I enjoy my own company, which I didn't when I was younger for some reason.

And I want to love my boys and my husband as much as I can so that when I'm gone, they can still feel my love. My husband and I have been married for twenty-three years, and when I leave this world or he does, we'll guide each other out. There's something really beautiful in that. People fear death or things about getting older, but I think we can make gentle shifts to see the beauty in it."

Who do you admire and look up to for how they're aging?
"I love Jane Fonda. She's so smart and passionate. She's 85 and still going strong with her film career and what she does for the environment. Sometimes people say, 'But look at all the work she's had done.' That's her right, and it doesn't make her any less. It's the same thing as when women give birth and people ask, 'Did you have a C-section? Vaginal birth? An epidural?' It doesn't matter. That's how I feel about cosmetic procedures. Do I personally like

it? No, I don't. But if I tried it and it worked, maybe I would have a different view. It's not my thing, but everyone should do what makes them comfortable."

Agreed! Thank you for this chat, Helen. Is there anything else you want to share with* The Glow Code *readers?

"Whatever your struggles are now, in your forties, take the time to look at them and work through them. Because whatever is holding you back now will be heightened. Do you fear getting old and being invisible? Do you fear gaining weight or having wrinkles? Look at why that is, work on it, and start to heal it so you can move forward with more grace. And take good care of yourself, because without your health, you have nothing. Nurture your body, listen to it, and give it what it needs. And last, know that much of the stuff we worry about with aging doesn't happen, so just let it go."

Ashton Applewhite

Ashton Applewhite is an award-winning writer, a full-time activist, and one seriously cool chick. I can confirm the last thing because I had the pleasure of speaking with her in May 2023 after Helen kindly introduced us. As for the previous two, well, Ashton's work speaks for itself.

She started to write seriously in her forties—an act precipitated by deciding she had to end her marriage while raising two young kids. When she found out two-thirds of divorces in the U.S. are initiated by women, and always have been, she paused to wonder why more people didn't know that or appreciate the implications. "We assume 98 percent of divorces are guys dumping their sad, washed-up wives—versions like me—for fertile, trophy versions," she told me from her home in Brooklyn. "I got angry so few people knew these things about marriage. And they don't know these things because we live in a sexist, misogynist, patriarchal society." Cue Ashton writing her first book, *Cutting Loose: Why Women Who End Their Marriages Do So Well.*

A similar process started her second book, *This Chair Rocks: A Manifesto Against Ageism*. As she explains on her website, thischairrocks.com, ageism is stereotyping and discriminating based on a person's age. While she writes about ageism cutting both ways, she acknowledges older people, or "olders" as she calls them, bear the brunt of it. Veering into older territory herself, Ashton wrote a book to dismantle the many myths about aging and rally the troops on a pro-aging crusade. "I just got so riled up that we are all, especially women, so hostage to this fucked-up narrative that makes us feel like pieces of shit. Why are we hostage to it? Why do we buy into it?"

She doesn't, at least not anymore.

Because as Ashton, who's now in her early seventies, discovered while researching her book, the fears she once had about aging were not only unfounded, they were incorrect. Though it's deeply human to fear many changes as we age, "only two unwelcome ones are inevitable: We'll lose people we've known all our lives, and some part of our bodies will fall apart," she wrote. "These changes are natural. But we live in a culture that has yet to develop the language and tools to help us deal with them."

Ashton is striving to change the language and culture, to empower people of all ages to reject ageism, which is, at its core, "a prejudice against our own future selves." Here's a glimpse into the conversation we had about her efforts, her work, and her life.

Let's start with a hard-hitting question: Have you seen Martha Stewart on the cover of* Sports Illustrated*?

"As a rule, I don't comment on women's appearances, but I will say I wish Martha didn't pin anti-aging cream because *that* is toxic. But I think it's fantastic she's out there as a sexual being at 80. Yes, she's an outlier, and yes, she's protected by enormous class and race privilege. Still, representation matters. And if people don't like her on the cover, it has more to do with misogyny and ageism, our own internalized stuff. And because the most vicious form of vitriol in this context is aimed at older women, go Martha!"

I've been reading and loving* This Chair Rocks. *I actually feel emotional talking to you because your pro-aging message is firing me up. What are some of the biggest surprises you had while writing your book?
"The biggest surprises happened very early on, like learning about the U-curve of happiness that says people are happiest at the beginnings and ends of their lives and that older people have better rates of mental health. Because I just assumed it was all going to suck, and another thing that was going to make it *super* suck was that you got closer to death. But turns out the longer people live, the less they fear dying. I don't know that I fear it less. I turned 70 last year, and it was a big number. It made me think about how much runway I have left. But I am a pragmatist and a de facto social scientist, and I'm scrupulously careful about my data. So, it was all a surprise to learn these things. And as I say about my book, you cannot read it and not feel better about the years ahead."

An idea you share that hit me so hard is that ageism is a prejudice against our own future selves, a denial that we will get old, that we* are *aging.
"Yes, all prejudice requires an 'Other.' And anyone who thinks hard about ageism realizes the 'Other' is not the white supremacist down the block or the person from the country across the way, it is your own future self.

Another slight problem with that framing is it's only in terms of prejudice against older people. And it's important to acknowledge that ageism is any judgment based on age, and younger people do experience a lot of it but, of course, olders experience more of it.

And it is like a distancing from your own self. Self-loathing is a big part of it. I mean, all this shit about anti-aging as wellness? Self-loathing is not well. It does not promote wellness."

How do you suggest parents speak to their kids about aging? How do we model good age behavior for the next generation?
"My first reaction is that we should not make age any different from how we talk about race or gender or any other identifier. In fact, I would say age is easier because we are *all* aging. And if you're not sure what the right thing to say is, ask and listen. When we put age or sex or race on the table as a topic, we can talk about how we're all learning together. That is the starting point.

But in the specific context of age, we live in a culture bombarding us with messages that aging is awful and shameful. So, the first step is to examine your own attitudes toward age and aging and think about how you use the words 'old' and 'young' and how you refer to your own age. Do you talk about and model age as a valuable, interesting component of identity as human beings, along with whether we like nachos or we're from Ukraine?

Age is a part of us, and it is a powerful, important part of our identity, but it's not better to be older. It's not better to be younger. There are good and bad aspects, in terms of how the world supports us and abandons us, about every age."

You have said making a friend a lot older or younger is one of the most powerful acts against ageism. I'm assuming you have friends that are both?
"Yes. We think that we won't have things in common with people who aren't our age, but aside from the occasional cultural reference, it's not a good reason to assume you will or won't like somebody.

In my early forties, my partner and I went to a huge electronic dance club and met this group of younger people, including a woman I would describe as one of my very closest friends. She's twenty years younger than I am and now has a son who's the same age as my grandson. They just visited, so we had a dance party in the house. Her son was watching us clear out the furniture for the party, and he said to me, 'Are you still going to be alive enough to go to these parties when I'm old?'

Maybe other people would be put off or think that's rude, but that's the kind of straightforward question you can get when age and death are not fraught. I said to him, 'That is such a good question! And yes, I think so. I'm not sure, but let's see what we can do.'"

I love that. Thank you, Ashton! Is there anything else you'd be passionate about sharing with women navigating midlife?

"It's incredibly important for women of all ages to come together. If more older women had younger women friends, we would be reminded of how hard it is to be young. But older women often resent younger women and want to distance themselves because they think being around younger women will make them look old. And you know what? You *will* look older than they are. But if you're pinning your value on that, you're already so vulnerable. And if more younger women were friends with older women, they would see how age is this time of fantastic power and authenticity. And friendships, in general, are crucial. Having friends of all ages enriches you, just like having friends who are different from you in every way."

Be sure to check out the Coming into Focus podcast from April 11, 2023. Helen interviews Ashton, and it's a fantastic conversation.

Nadia Hrkac

Nadia Hrkac is a Toronto-based specialty foods importer, a registered holistic nutritionist, and—how fortunate for me—my dear, close friend. We met twenty years ago when I studied journalism in Toronto and dated her brother's good friend. He and I broke up, but Nadia and I are forever. Though we don't live in the same city anymore, we stay in touch. We talk. We message. And we travel together when we can.

At 53, Nadia is many things—proudly single, an entrepreneur, a loving aunt, a world adventurer. To me, and at ten years my senior, she is a real-life example of a woman aging with ease and confidence, a glorious being who feels comfortable in her skin. Our conversations over the years have helped shape my feelings about aging, encouraged me to embrace my lines and wrinkles, and inspired me to age with pride. Just spending time in her orbit makes me excited about the years ahead.

One of our many chats stands out because it sparked deep reflection on what I want for myself as I age. We were sitting on the patio of a Mexican restaurant in Toronto when Nadia told me why she was choosing to forego Botox and fillers, despite feeling like an outlier among women her age. She eventually shared the same reason on Instagram when I asked my followers how they felt about cosmetic procedures to "fix" their wrinkles and lines: "Never had anything done as I truly believe in aging gracefully and naturally. Not against it but want to embrace looking the way nature intended without the pressure of preserving the way we looked at a certain age. Being your true, authentic self is liberating."

Nadia's words and, most importantly, her actions have profoundly affected me. It's only fitting I end this chapter, and this book, with her. The following is a bit of the conversation we had in July 2023.

As you know, I have always admired how you embrace aging. Where do your views on aging come from?

"When I was in my early thirties, the age it seems when everyone starts panicking about getting older, I dated a great guy named Scott. And I remember saying to him, 'My biggest fear is ending up old and alone.' He convinced me to watch a documentary called "Age Is No Barrier" and—I get goosebumps thinking about this—it changed the course of my life. The film shows a group of seniors getting together at a gym to do gymnastics, and watching it alleviated 80 to 90 percent of my fear. I realized that fear is such an illusion and, even if you're alone, getting old doesn't have to be scary if you're healthy and take care of yourself."

You can watch "Age Is No Barrier," a 24-minute documentary released in 1989, for free on the National Film Board of Canada website.

That's amazing, and I know you prioritize self-care. What does your everyday routine look like?

"I take good care of my skin, and I've had to start doing more than just wearing natural skincare because I'm getting older. I do a clay mask at least once a week and have a peel from a professional skincare line. And one of my favorite things is something called AlkaBath from Dr. P. Jentschura, a German biochemist and natural doctor who basically takes Epsom salts to a Porsche level. I also have a green juice every day, and I prioritize sleep. All these little things make me feel super, super happy."

Where does your confidence come from, and has it changed as you age?

"There was a side of me that wasn't confident when I was younger, and I know that because I attracted a certain type of guy. I guess I was seeking some type of validation, or I wanted to fix them, whatever it was. But I'm becoming more naturally confident as I age because of my knowledge, work experience, and just knowing I can be okay alone. And having discipline is a confidence-builder, too. Even when I'm not feeling well or I'm tired, I can make myself a healthy meal or go accomplish something, and that makes me feel good."

What excites you most about the years ahead?

"This might sound lame, but my business. It's what brings me the most joy in life. I'm not saying it's the same as having a child, but it's kind of similar! It's like when someone interviewed Jennifer Aniston and mentioned she's not a mom. She said, 'Well, I've birthed many things.' I feel like I birthed my business, and there's no better feeling than watching it grow."

Speaking of celebrities, who do you admire for how they're approaching aging?

"Kate Winslet is my number one, hands down, but there are others. Cameron Diaz said she tried Botox and didn't like it because she didn't look like herself anymore. She said, 'I'd rather see my face aging than a face that doesn't belong to me at all.' And I'm so glad she said that because it's how I feel. I mean, never say never, and I'm not vehemently preaching against it, but because I'm so into natural health, it goes against who I am.

There's something so freeing about being comfortable with your age and just accepting it. But there's this panic that seems to be inflicted on women. We are changing as we age because we're *supposed* to be changing, and it's natural to be changing physically because we're evolving as women."

What advice would you share with younger women about how we can embrace this aging thing?

"Don't panic! [*She laughs.]* That's my joke. The main thing I'd say is do things for yourself. We're all different, so do things that boost your confidence level because those things will prevent you from going down a rabbit hole. For me, it's cooking, being healthy, working out, and feeding my business. Every woman has to build confidence her own way, and there are no shortcuts. No one else can do it for you. But the effort is worth it. Aging is all about how you feel on the inside."

Thank you, Nadia. I love you to pieces.

And, finally, thank you to *all* the women in my world—friends, family members, colleagues, and more—for inspiring me as we tackle this whole aging thing together. I treasure every one of you.

CONCLUSION

THOUGH MY *GLOW CODE* EXPERIMENT HAS ENDED, YOURS IS JUST beginning. And I have many hopes for you, my dear reader.

I hope you feel informed, encouraged, and inspired.

I hope you don't feel stressed or overwhelmed. I've thrown a lot at you in this book, but please consider it an advice buffet, a choose-your-own-adventure situation. Enact change where it makes sense for you. Pick your action items based on your interest, capacity, and, most importantly, the priorities that will lead you to become the older woman you want to be. And if you do nothing else but start thinking about who you want to become as you age, then you're already off to a good start.

Most importantly, I hope you feel empowered to enact simple, effective changes to boost your health, happiness, and well-being. As your humble guide and guinea pig, I know it's possible. The advice in this book works. At this very moment, I'm sipping my protein coffee and plan to break from writing in half an hour for a HIRT workout. Later this afternoon, I'll meditate for ten minutes. And tonight, while watching a movie with my kids, I'll pull out my knitting to work on my dress. The tips and insights in this book have improved the quality and depth of my everyday life, and I have no doubt the benefits will continue to play out as I age.

When I set out to write this book, I was hunting for tips and advice to help us gals feel great and age well now, through midlife, and beyond. I found those, but I unearthed much more. Some key learnings and *aha* moments I've had along the way have shifted my thinking on what it means to age well and helped refine my priorities accordingly. Here they are, shaped into one final cheat sheet.

THE CHEAT SHEET

- **Embrace the notion that less is more (except for sleep).** The moment I realized less is more, be it with my fitness regime, skincare routine, or meditation requirements, I breathed a sigh of relief. Many of the most impactful changes I've made have involved scaling back on something in my life or adding the bare minimum of something else. Small tweaks can have big impacts, my friends, and that's so encouraging.
- **Choose consistency over perfection, always.** Whether it's how I'm exercising, managing my bad habits, or even interacting with loved ones, I'm aiming for consistency over perfection in all areas of my life. I'm so done with the idea of having perfect homes, perfect bodies, perfect relationships, perfect anything, and I hope you are, too. Consistency—glorious, boring consistency—is the key.
- **Make peace with your age.** When body-image coach Summer Innanen told me women don't have to love their bodies—we should aim for body neutrality instead—I had an epiphany: What if we extended that same philosophy to our age? It may be too much to ask me, you, or any woman to *love* our age, especially as we become "olders" and face aspects that are harder to embrace. Being age neutral, however, is liberating. Age does not define us, just as our bodies do not.
- **Aging well means living well, so let's live on our own terms.** Ashton Applewhite, the writer and activist leading the fight against ageism, talks about how aging just means living. It's a simple but powerful reminder. Because it

> means if we want to age well, we must live well. And every woman's path will be different, her goals and priorities unique. My idea of living and aging well will differ from yours. There is no right or successful way to do it, so let's live authentically, making choices that bring us closer to ourselves and the women we hope to become.

One last thought. Though I'm striving to make the most of these years—optimizing everything from my health and well-being to my relationships and daily routines—I now remind myself, especially on my hardest days, that I am good enough. No matter what. At any age. As I recently saw someone post on Instagram, "The real glow up is when you stop waiting to turn into some perfect version of yourself and consciously enjoy being who you are in the present."

That's such a peaceful way to think about aging. I don't want to mourn the loss of who I once was or what I looked like, nor do I want to worry about what the future will bring. I want to feel great, appreciate each day, and fully embrace this and every stage of my life. Ultimately, I'm on a mission to age gratefully, and I hope you feel the same. Because I believe if we can be thankful for every passing year of our wondrous lives, we will unleash a glow—a radiance grounded in gratitude—that lasts a lifetime.

Thank you for joining me on this journey, and please email me anytime at hello@michelle-mcivor.com to share your thoughts and experiences as you put this cheat sheet to work in your life. I'd love to hear from you.

Here's to us all living and aging well.

ACKNOWLEDGMENTS

First and foremost, thank you to my incredible agent Kathryn Willms, who has believed in me from the day she read my two-sentence pitch for this book. Kathryn, I could not have done this without you, nor would I have wanted to. Thank you for your guidance, brilliant feedback, and friendship. I am beyond lucky you're in my corner.

I am proud to be represented by The Rights Factory and grateful to our leader Sam Hiyate for connecting me with Kathryn and championing my book from the beginning. Thank you, Sam. Special shoutout to Claire Cavanagh for being one of my first readers and letting me know which lines made her laugh out loud (a confidence boost I desperately needed). And thank you to Gillian Chapman for helping me with marketing research for my book at the eleventh hour. You were a lifesaver.

Huge thanks to Suzanne Staszak-Silva for acquiring my book for Rowman & Littlefield and my fantastic publishing team for bringing *The Glow Code* to life, especially Jacqueline Flynn, Joanna Wattenberg, Neil Cotterill, Amy Paradysz, Anna Keyser, Susan Hershberg, and Veronica Dove. Thank you for everything.

I must express my heartfelt gratitude (again) to my interviewees for sharing their wisdom with me and my readers. Though most of the people I spoke with are listed at the front of the book and quoted throughout, I also want to thank several women who inspired my writing, specifically Lucky Bromhead, Michelle

Segar, Tish Duffy, Chloe Szcyglowski, Gill Gazdic, and Keri-Leigh Cassidy. You are all divine beings.

Arranging more than forty interviews was no small task, and I could not have done it alone. I am forever indebted to the people in my world who connected me with the people in their worlds for interviews or pointed me in the right direction, namely John Berardi, Adam Grant, Rida Abboud, Lyle Reimer, Lana Rogers, Steve Mesler, Marie Claire Bourque, and Gwendolyn Richards. Thank you, all. (I'm positive I'm missing people on this list, so my deepest apologies to anyone I haven't named.)

And thanks to many of my interviewees who, at the end of our chats, said something like, "Have you thought of speaking with . . ." and then sent email introductions on my behalf to their colleagues. An extra-special thank-you to Helen Tansey, who not only agreed to be interviewed and then introduced me to Ashton Applewhite but generously offered to take my author photo for the book. Spending time with you was magical, Helen.

Thank you to my beloved friends and fellow journalists Christina Frangou and Malwina Gudowska for your sublime friendship and support in all things writing. I appreciate you so much.

Natalie MacLean and Christine Gibson, thank you for sharing your book-publishing experiences to help me navigate mine.

And speaking of publishing, I extend major thanks to Tim Ferriss, who offered to use his social media platforms to spread the word about *The Glow Code* on my publication date. You're the best, Tim.

I'd be remiss not to thank David Hayes, who taught me how to be a freelance magazine writer during my final semester of journalism school in 2005. Thank you for nudging me along my writing path, David.

I am fortunate to have exceptional friends whose awesomeness kept me afloat while in the book-writing weeds. Thank you from the bottom of my heart to Samantha Descoteaux-Kahane, Jennifer Rende, Anna Palmiere, Haithem Elkadiki, Sarah Giani,

Kaysi Fagan, and Andrée Roberts for always checking in to see how the writing was going, offering ideas, and encouraging me over a glass or two of rosé. I don't know what I'd do without you.

To the McIvor family, thank you for your love. My dear brother-in-law Colin passed away in April 2022 while I was writing this book, and his memory inspires me daily. What a blessing to have had you in my life, Colin.

There isn't a thank-you massive enough for my parents, Bonnie and Daniel Magnan, who instilled my love of reading and writing, cut out every newspaper and magazine article I ever wrote, and never failed to ask how the book was coming along. Thank you for your unwavering belief in me, Mom and Dad, and your love. And to my brother, Brent Magnan, thank you for always showing up for me in ways big and small. I feel so lucky to have a brother who is also one of my closest friends.

Finally, thank you to my little family, my greatest joy. Hudson and Marlowe, you are my sunshine, and I am incredibly proud to be your mom. To Cameron, the best husband a gal could ask for, thank you for your unending support, devotion, and belief that I would handle our story with care. Not many people would receive the draft of a chapter with details about their sex life and then wait two weeks to read it, but you did—and then gave it a glowing review. I love your self-assuredness, not to mention your wit and intelligence.

I am eternally grateful for you, Cam, Hudson, and Marlowe, and the beautiful life we share.

INDEX

Note italicized pages references indicate illustrations

ABOUT THE AUTHOR

Michelle McIvor is a journalist on a mission to age gratefully. A former health and wellness columnist with the *Calgary Herald*, her writing has appeared in *Maclean's*, *Chatelaine*, *Best Health*, and *AskMen*, among other publications. Michelle has also ghostwritten two books, including the #1 Canadian bestseller *Forever Terry: A Legacy in Letters*. She lives in Calgary, Alberta, with her husband and two kids.